ROOTLINES

ROOTLINES

A Memoir

RIKKI WEST

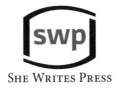

SHE WRITES PRESS

Published 2020
Printed in the United States of America
ISBN: 978-1-63152-753-1
ISBN: 978-1-63152-754-8
Library of Congress Control Number: 2020905479

For information, address:
She Writes Press
1569 Solano Ave #546
Berkeley, CA 94707

She Writes Press is a division of SparkPoint Studio, LLC.

All company and/or product names may be trade names, logos, trademarks, and/or registered trademarks and are the property of their respective owners.

Names and identifying characteristics have been changed to protect the privacy of certain individuals. "Mountainware" is a fictional name for an actual technology company.

For Rosemary Biritz and Dick West

CONTENTS

THE BELL TOLLS

GRAPPLING

FIGHT FOR MYSELF

MAGIC MARKERS

CHEMO

TRIALS

TRANSPLANT

RECOVERY

THRIVING

INTRODUCTION

A person goes on a pilgrimage. She's on foot and wearing good boots. She carries a well-supplied backpack and a flat-brimmed sun hat but no compass. No extra stuff—no camera, walking staff, or binoculars. She could be walking anywhere, from Colorado to New Zealand, when she encounters a wizened old neighbor at the intersection of any two roads.

Neighbor: Greetings, friend. Where are you headed?

Wanderer: I am on pilgrimage.

Neighbor: How unusual. What are you seeking on your pilgrimage?

Wanderer: I don't know.

Neighbor: Good. Not knowing is most intimate.

This story is told as Case #20 in the collection of koans known as *The Book of Equanimity*. It raises questions. Who is that benevolent neighbor out there, checking on the welfare of wanderers? That's helpful! Can you actually expect the world to support you if you embark on such a quest? And this wanderer—what's up with her?

What does she mean by *pilgrimage*? How could she set out without knowing where she's going or what she's seeking, while exposing herself to the elements and all the wild unknown?

But then, come to think of it, all of us got launched into life without knowing. Without getting the chance to ask any questions, we just showed up around the age of two or three, trying to get along. Not knowing.

Though we aren't all on a pilgrimage, are we? Making a commitment like that is a serious choice, and a courageous one. You have to want it. The Seeker sets out on her wayfaring with intent. She pursues something unfamiliar, toward which she feels a vague pull, a leftwise attraction. Journeying on her own two feet, she embarks alone, looking for something she hasn't seen and trusting that more will be revealed. Yet when asked why she is on this pilgrimage, one that we imagine she intends to take with all her beating heart, she doesn't know.

She doesn't know? You can venture into the dark on just some gutsy inkling? That's interesting. She's no fool; she is not wandering aimlessly through life, waiting for someone to rescue her. "Not knowing" suggests she is open to genuine insights, that she has a mind that's willing to suspend comforting explanations. She's interested in something she *doesn't* know everything about. She's going to pry into what's really going on in any moment. Who is here? What's arising right now? What possibilities are present?

There's a hidden dark side here. How often does the heroine gambol into the dark woods to encounter something easy and delicious, like vanilla pudding? No one is saying it aloud, but our intrepid friend is going to walk into a few sandstorms—we can count on it. Yet the supportive elder approves, giving no warning. "Good approach. Most intimate."

PROLOGUE

Santa Cruz Mountains
August 2016

I am fighting for myself. The other guy is trying to hit me in the face, and I am trying to avoid that. But I am not fighting *against* him as much as I am fighting *for* me. Every aspect of me.

His jab lands repeatedly, and I feel ridiculed. I'm slipping correctly, aren't I? Isn't this what we practiced in class? I pivot. I keep my jab out there. I'm teeping—the front kick version of a jab—but he keeps landing. Bam-bam. I'm glad I got the deluxe helmet with extra cheek pads. I flip a double jab and step out, right into the cross. There's the bell—relief. Sweat is pouring down both of our faces. We have one minute before the next round of sparring. Our hearts are hammering because three minutes is a long time to face somebody whose life is focused on hitting and kicking you. I'm frustrated; I want to move faster. Get my legs under me and, for god's sake, block the right body kick. And I'm angry; his jab was dominating, and I hate being dominated. I reacted and started swinging wild and got a cross to the head for my foolishness. Now I need to regain my equanimity. I'm breathing through my nose to tell my brain I'm not panicking, everything is fine, keep executing. Bell!

I touch gloves with a woman about my size. Everything starts out fine: I catch a few jabs; she slips mine and lands a front kick. Why didn't I block? My mind drifts, and, pop! Something hits me in the face. Where was I? Pivot, teep, right kick. Relax. Bam-bam-bam at me, and I'm batting it away when two kicks land, bap-bap, lightly, on my arm just below the shoulder. I'm wiped out, my spirits sag, but no time for being a sad sack because we have 2:30 left to spar and I've got to get it going here.

Muay Thai demands physical courage. That's one reason I'm fighting. Self-respect is another. And the ability to regain my serenity. And confidence.

The workouts have reshaped my body. I've got shoulders and calves that my younger body never met. I've learned to absorb the jarring when a strike connects, so I don't lose focus. This training has made my whole body less fearful of aggression. That means it doesn't dump a load of cortisol into my blood and freeze me with fear before it's really necessary. It means my body trusts itself to handle a lot more before it starts to worry.

After you practice a move a thousand times, your body knows that move. The happy surprise is how quickly your body learns to choose good moves that deal with the entire situation. It can see a strike coming and raise a block before you even notice. Everyone who does a sport or plays an instrument or performs a thousand other physical arts relies on the penetrating intelligence of the body. Mine knows how to read a situation and orchestrate a complete response while my conscious mind is still trying to snap out of indignation that I just got tagged again.

The courage I'm seeking entails trusting the intelligence of my body. I want courage to confront challenges in family life. I want serenity to deal with grief and memories of my mother. I would enjoy more robust confidence and the feeling of ease and power that comes from a strong core. It will turn out that I will need all that before the end of summer 2016: trust, courage, serenity, confidence, and power.

The next morning, I receive an email from my older sister, Linda, saying her indolent follicular lymphoma, quiet for five or six years, has transformed to diffuse large B-cell lymphoma (DLBCL). The deformed B cells have clogged into tumors. There is no known chemo that can eliminate them. The tumors are tangled in her intestines and pressing a ureter. She has been given a prognosis of a painful though fairly rapid death. There is one iffy option for people with deadly blood cancers like this: vigorous chemotherapy to destroy the bone marrow and its stem cells, followed by a stem cell transplant.

When you deal with a terminal diagnosis, you think about the quality of life you will have after treatment. In the case of transplants, that depends on finding a highly matched donor, because innumerable complications arise from minor mismatches. The most likely, though still unlikely, place to find a good match is among your siblings. Alas, we two younger sisters, Elizabeth and I, are more than two decades over the age limit for donors, Linda writes.

Why am I hearing of this just now? My mind races. Has she been in pain? Did she say *death*? And she's just telling me?

Within seconds after that email dings my mailbox, mind still racing, I get Linda on the phone. We haven't spoken in months. "Stuff and nonsense," I tell her. "I am healthy and strong. I'll get tested." Linda bursts into tears, really rare for her. Linda has self-possession; Linda has dignity. I am much more likely to embarrass everyone with my Hallmark crying, while she is usually all business or all laughter. But we're way past personality types today.

Linda's aggressive lymphoma produces malformed B cells that look like dropped scoops of ice cream instead of marbles. B cells are magical cells from the immune system. Most cells have a firm library of DNA templates for the proteins they will build during their lives. B cells have the rare gift of being able to alter their own DNA templates, which means they have special power to fight disease. They reprogram their own genetics to build specific proteins that find and help kill invading bacteria and viruses. Without them, you're practically dead after the first sneeze. A simple cold virus will take over like scutch grass, opening the way for a deadly bacterial invasion. With no ability to mount an immune response, your body has a slim chance of surviving in the world. Think of the care we take with newborn babies while their immune systems develop.

If B cells are deformed, as they are in DLBCL, they clog up in nodules, building tumors that block metabolic functions. So you're dead from that anyway. The best-case scenario is to destroy the entire blood and lymph production system from the ground up and rebuild it with new genetics. The new genetics have to be very close to the original.

To find a donor, you search on registries like Be The Match, but your best chance for a good match—about 25 percent—is a sibling. Despite being way past prime donating age, I happen to be in the unequivocally healthiest state I have ever been in, thanks to years of steadily tougher workouts and training for sparring sessions. My bone marrow, source of stem cells, is primed for high-volume manufacturing because it is already supplying stem cells to build the new muscle, tendon, and blood vessels my workouts demand. Although I am old, I am a perfect potential donor.

But Linda has been afraid, or too angry, or too obstinate to tell me about her prognosis and her needs. We stopped speaking back in April after a huge fight. Our mother was very ill. My stepfather, Hank, died suddenly in March, and we were struggling with how to provide care for Mom. We crossed lines. I told Linda never to speak to me again, and she was sticking with it to the death. That's what it is like to be Hungarian, my uncle Matt would say. Or trapped in self-defeating, unconscious patterns, you could say about both of us. Linda resigned herself to death from this goddamn tumor, rather than ask me for help, all because I was so affronted that I wanted to cut her out of my life, for life. That is the kind of dangerous nonsense unconscious patterns can do to you.

Then, in June, Mom died. Now, in August, tumors show up in Linda's positron-emission tomography (PET) scan. This is getting too real. We have no room for petty squabbles, yet hurt feelings are lying around like wounded Heffalumps. Who can even remember what we fought over? Perhaps I was as egocentric, self-centered, and blathering as she said. Perhaps I wasn't but she believed I was. So what? Who cares? I guess she doesn't have to like me for me to love her. One of us is dying. One of us might save her life. Who are we, either of us, when we drop the posturing? A couple of fragile, vulnerable, living beings who want to know what happens tomorrow.

"Don't give up yet, Linda," I say. "How do I get tested? What should I do?"

"Oh! Oh, thank you. I . . . but I have to go." Flustered, she wants to hang up. "I'll call you back; let me find out and call you back later. Thank you, Rikki." I hear her tears as she disconnects. I sit with phone in hand, staring at my desk.

My desk is a sheet of worried tin wrapped around plywood set on a wooden frame about thigh height. Stacks of notebooks and note cards splash across it; loose lined sheets of yellow or white, folded, marked in tumbling blue lines or penciled with numbered lists. Mechanical pencils, fiber-tipped pens, and scissors jut up from a blue ceramic mug; next to it, a leather penholder displays my five working fountain pens. The desiccated, smoky scent of old coffee floats over my empty cup. Notes on stickies; a to-do list. Here is a sheet torn from an essay book with three writing tips I gleaned from reading Tom Franklin. Here is a bill for two white screen door–closer kits. My throat has narrowed to a thin straw. Out the window, a cornucopia of evergreen: juniper, redwood, pine, cypress. The wild grasses and thistle have grown too high; we will need to mow soon. This time of year, they are a fire hazard.

I will always have Linda's back, I think. *Doesn't she know that? Don't we have each other's backs?*

And really, the only reason I can have her back this time is a miracle. For some reason I had become a Muay Thai kickboxer, which I started as a way to cope with work stress just three years before.

THE BELL TOLLS

UNEXPECTED GUIDE

MountainWare
Spring 2013

"Just ask for a moment to compose yourself," my boss at MountainWare says.

"We've discussed this; you know I can't do networking," I tell him. We are standing in my window office in Building C at MountainWare. I am so frustrated with this man, I just want to bang my head against the whiteboard and make it all go away. "OS and SysOps are my background. I just spent two years embedded with those guys. You pull me out now, you end my career here." My head hurts.

Pierre shrugs. "I want to see how Anish handles SysOps. You can work with Greg in Networking." He sits on the edge of my filing cabinet, watching me with a slight sneer—or is it just the way his lips fall? Intense blue eyes pock his boyish, fleshy face.

"Excuse me. I am taking a moment." I walk, head up, through my door, into the hall, step by step, approaching the relative safety of the ladies' room. I plop down in the breastfeeding chair in the infant room and do some deep breathing. I am fighting for my job here. At sixty-two, I know this is most likely my last, and I want to keep it as long as possible. My boss is reassigning me to work with the

Networking team, pulling me off the SysOps team, where I've racked up a few wins. I will probably die in Networking. Pierre is ambitiously working to expand his portfolio. To do this, he needs technical security engineers, but his promised hiring budget has been cut. So he plans to lay off his nontechnical staff to get some head count he can use on his scheme. One of the steps in the plan is for me to face-plant in Networking. Plus, Pierre has a bone to pick with me. In a recent argument with his boss, he lost. The boss sided with me, and now I'm paying for that momentary pleasure.

The Networking team poses a technical challenge for me. In addition, most of my work would be with the team in India; few of the Networking security engineers are in the United States. That means late nights and early mornings, working from home, and short days at the office. I didn't object to that; it's standard operating procedure for the fifty-hour international workweek in high tech, and I'm willing to do almost anything. What I mind is being placed intentionally in a position to fail because my skill set doesn't match the assignment. Pierre is new to his job; his predecessor, who hired me, had a policy of using people's strengths. She promised to keep me in SysOps, where I have some strength.

Damn you, Pierre, I say to myself in the privacy of the nursing chair. *It's just like Chuck at Nokia, but this time I can see it happening. You're using us not for the real mission of our group, but for your personal gain.*

Thirty years. I've been in this industry that long, and this sadly prosaic management behavior still upsets me. *OK,* I tell myself, *you're probably in the grip of a little work-related PTSD.* It's true; work distress has plagued me since a layoff at Nokia in 2001. *Just work your butt off, and you can make it come together.* I commit myself to the Networking assignment. I will not let this man take me down. But the Nokia ordeal, and the terrible period of loss that followed, reverberate in my mind.

Nokia, April 2001

Anyone who was in high tech during the dot-com bust at the turn of the century has a few dramatic experiences to tell their friends about, but layoffs at Nokia in 2001 shook me up. I was the director of engineering and site manager of the Nokia office in Scotts Valley, California. One spring morning, coffee in hand, I was in my office, gathering papers for a meeting that would start in a few minutes. A human resources representative appeared at the door with my boss, Chuck. Chuck was tall, and his figure filled the door. I suddenly felt trapped. They both came into my office and told *me* to sit down, rather than asking if *they* could.

"What meeting were you going to?" Chuck said. I answered; then he said, "You're not going to any more meetings. You're suspended, pending an investigation of how you handled this company memo," he said, putting a copy on the table. I stared at it without comprehending it at all. "Security is on the way to escort you out of the building."

I couldn't hear anything except the sound of a waterfall. I don't recall any further conversation. A security officer arrived, and I was permitted to gather my stuff. He then escorted me out of my office, down the hallway, to the elevator, to the lobby, and out of the building. Our parade went past the offices and windows of my staff and the other managers at our site. I had to walk across the campus parking lot to my car, while the windows of my group's offices and conference rooms gaped down at my lonely Honda Civic.

An investigation was supposed to follow, but in the end Nokia simply laid me off with the rest when they closed the site. I was just over fifty years old. For the rest of my career, I would have the background suspicion that my boss was collecting excuses to fire me. A relatively harmless question like "What time did you leave last night?" would leave my palms sweating.

The story got around the then-small world of Silicon Valley. Plus, the dot-com bust wiped out many companies, and jobless talent flooded the market. It took me years to get another position and my feet back on the ground. I tapped unknown reserves of courage to start fresh every day. I had a young daughter to care for, and she gave me strength.

A single parent, I intended from the start to be the sole provider and caregiver for my daughter, Lauren Magnolia, who before junior high school was already a vegetarian. In fifth grade, she learned how animals were treated in our agricultural practices and immediately swore off meat. We had to reorganize our kitchen to accommodate her ethics, and it was only a few years before I converted to join her. Though her father, Nick, a dear friend, passed away when she was not yet two, his partner, Daddy Robert, stayed in Lauren's life as her dad. But he did not share financial responsibilities with me. I was on my own.

I was facing one of the scariest challenges of being a single parent—the loss of income. There seemed nowhere to turn. I got stuck in a defeating cycle of self-condemnation. My inner strength was bewilderingly inaccessible to me. I was over an edge. I attacked myself for my choices, my skills, my limitations, my character. *You're a fucking idiot*, I said. *Why don't you know another profession? Why can't you learn to code?* I got stuck in a bad rut.

I resented that things had gone this way, when they should have gone differently. This was the wrong life. *What happened? What did I do wrong? What's wrong with me?* I was sure that some mistake I had made was the source of the trouble. And that thought—that a mistake had been made somewhere—was the incorrect thought, driven by an unconscious pattern, that kept me from confronting what I could actually do about the whole situation. I just kept making myself collapse under the weight of *What did I do wrong?* and *I don't know what to do.* The unconscious pattern was this: *You made mistakes because you are an idiot, you are broken, and you will always fail.*

The sixteenth-century Hindu mystic poet Mirabai wrote, "Without the energy that lifts mountains, how am I to live?" Some kind of energy was not filling me. The energy that lifts mountains was blocked in me. You wake up (a friend once put it) with your head about three feet below street level. It's a struggle to get up to the ground floor. That is a terrifying, dark place. I took myself to a yoga center where I could meditate, chant, and study with good people. There I found access to some of that elusive energy and ways to forgive the clawlike grip I had fastened on myself. I talked with people who understood me and read accounts of a dark night of the soul, which sounded a lot like what I was having. While I looked for work, I developed a daily meditation habit. I found ways to raise my spirits, and over time I came to respect myself for at least taking ownership of that crappy depression.

Hundreds of résumés and applications later, my brother-in-law called to offer me a part-time, contract, project management job. I snapped it up like it was the best thing I had ever heard—and it was! I had made it across the great Nokia Divide, and things began to turn around.

All of that happened a decade before MountainWare. I fought my way back from that slide into desperation and loss. I meditated my way through and, at some point, found the bottom. There, I heard my own voice calling out to me in my own heart. *If you are still there, showing up for yourself at the very bottom, you are someone you can count on.* After working myself out of that deep pit, I started to relate to myself in a friendlier way. From there began a slow return of my attention and energy to my own body and life in the present. In AA they call that a new freedom and a new happiness.

I've been putting my life back together, stone by stone. Lauren has graduated from college, with her hair tangled in dreadlocks, her spirit embedded in music, and her heart committed to social justice. We have made it through the start of higher education and all the teenage years. She is entering graduate school, as a strong, self-defining woman who is determined to live her values and keeps, as a constant companion, a gigantic dog, half wolf and half something that drools like a Swiss mountain dog. I have a decent project management position at MountainWare. I am in a good partner relationship that has withstood years and challenges. At this point, I am committed to fight for myself. It is my turn to find my personal power to choose and act. It is my turn for the freedom to thrive and to refresh, somehow, the willingness to keep generating love.

I am not going to let the past or Pierre or MountainWare dictate how my life unfolds. I am in it to win it.

Pierre threatens to fire some of us and actually carries it out. One Monday morning, we come in and find an empty workstation in a cubicle outside the window offices. An unplugged monitor sits next to a keyboard and mouse. Naked pushpins poke a corkboard, the whiteboard is wiped, and the computer is gone. One of us has disappeared over the weekend. It is pretty unnerving.

Tuesday morning, Pierre changes our one-on-one time because, he says, while patting his belly, he has scheduled workouts with a trainer at the gym. Ping! What a great idea! This is exactly what *I* need to cope with the stress he sparks. I am never going to have the discipline to work out on my own. However, if I pay a trainer, I will show up and do the work. And if Pierre can leave his desk to work out, so can I. I literally jog over to the company gym that minute, before I change my mind.

I arrive panting outside the locker rooms and find the manager at the front desk. I ask about fitness packages; there are options. Happily, I learn that everything is subsidized for MountainWare employees. I sign up with a trainer named Jake Timoteo. It is a smart move for my health and sanity, but it also sets me up to meet Linda's future stem cell needs. I don't understand this yet. Only in retrospect will I see how perfectly woven into the fabric of healing this opportunity is. As far as I know right now, I'm just trying to keep my job, minimize stress, stay sane.

My work with Jake makes me sweat and cry. We start slowly, with stretches, small weights, sit-ups. We cheer my little victories. Week by week, we challenge my body in the full range of fitness, including running, lifting, pulling, jumping, squatting, and all the other "-ings." He makes it lighthearted, and he always seems fearless in pushing me to another level that I am certain will produce the heart attack or torn ligament I fear. He teaches me how to stand up and walk it off.

Back at the office, Pierre continues pushing hard to expand his influence. Other ambitious men push back. Work sucks! I put my nose to the grindstone. I set up the Problem Report Review for 9:00 p.m. PST. We do the Hercules Project Scrum at 6:00 a.m. One-on-one discussions get scattered between 6:00 and 9:00 p.m., 5:00 and 10:00 a.m. Engineers on both sides of the world scramble through traffic and rearrange family plans, skipping dinners or working early. I track work items, get commitments from engineers, compile statistics, update the right databases, and generate reports. I make sure people have the information they need to make decisions, and I track actions to make sure we keep our commitments. I want to save my neck by getting real work done. I think if I try hard enough, at least it would be embarrassing for anyone to fire me for incompetence. People on my teams give me positive feedback.

I keep up the workouts because I like Jake and he makes me feel so successful. Each week we add reps or pounds or seconds. Each week I feel better and stronger. And my body is changing. Jake makes everything fun; all I have to do is whatever he tells me to do in that moment. I don't have to worry about the next thing, about how many or how much. I just have to execute.

"Are you ready to kick butt today, Rikki?"

"I am always ready, Jake!" You can get into a zone where your complaints stop—or, anyway, the volume goes way down.

Then one day he pulls out some boxing gloves and tells me about Thai kickboxing, called Muay Thai.

My father was a boxer in the army, so maybe I've come to this passion via Daddy. I remember his brown, creased, worn leather lace-up gloves, which I loved with singular fascination. Jake slips a pair of his black leather gloves onto my hands and fastens the Velcro straps. I feel a genuine thrill. He holds up focus mitts and shows me how to plant my feet for the jab.

"Pop it right in here," he calls out, holding up a mitt with his left. I muff my glove into his mitt. No pop. "Pop it! Right here!" Muff. Puff. I plant my feet. Pip. I snap my punch. Pop! Pop! Oh yeah, the jab hitting the mitt. Pop! Pop! It's kind of hot! It excites me; it's almost erotic, but happier. I want this thing, this Thai kickboxing. Since it is Jake, I know I have a chance. He can get me there. I will be able to do this Muay Thai, and oh, Lordy, that will be fun.

Things continue to fall apart at the office. Team members resign and move on. Of twenty-three people on the team when Pierre joined, in a few months only fifteen are left. I quit the MountainWare gym and sign up at Jake's fight club, KOA Fitness in Mountain View, where I train in Muay Thai four times a week. Did you know it can take years to perfect the jab?

When Pierre ignores my status reports, I do kicking drills. When seven more people quit, I hit the bag. When Pierre gives me a crummy review, I spar extra rounds. Why? Because it makes me outrageous and because it is life in my face and because it makes me into a warrior. And I look great and feel greater and have muscles that make me feel powerful. I love Muay Thai. Who knew it would also serve a greater good? When the time comes to save a life, it is astonishing that I, who prefers to sit around and read, will be so fit and strong.

My crisis at MountainWare peters out. I survive it! In the summer of 2015, Pierre quits, moving on to being a director of something in San Francisco. By the fall, there are just three of us left. I confront our director about the personnel management issues we experienced. Finally, in January 2016, the last two employees in the group quit and I get laid off. Free at last, I am a sixty-four-year-old kickboxer in training. I begin to think about signing up for a real amateur fight.

But I don't have much free time, as the year turns out to be a continual confrontation with the things that scare me most.

SUDDEN DECLINE

Pine Mountain Club
Mt. Pinos Area
Winter and Spring 2016

In February, out of the blue, my stepdad, Hank, is diagnosed with pancreatic cancer. He passes away within weeks. A tall, thin, composed man, he was in excellent physical and mental health until that moment. He bore the burden alone of caring for a less-than-healthy Mom. Suddenly Mom's care is in our hands, and she needs 24-7 assistance with basic life management. Linda and Elizabeth arrive within hours. I drive down from Santa Cruz to Pine Mountain Club the next day. The most immediate challenge is helping her understand what has happened. Dementia and mini-strokes have weakened her memory severely.

We have to tell her many times that Hank has passed. Each time is an agony; once was bad enough. Her world has become a corridor from the dining table to the bed to the bathroom. His world had shrunk to the size of hers. And, despite his near indifference to her at the end, she loved him in her desperate way. Life without him will be even worse for Mother, who cannot see, hear, remember, or move around much.

By this time, she's withdrawn profoundly from this world, a process that began many years ago. She and Hank, her second husband and probably second lover, retreated to their bespoke home in the San Emigdio Mountain forests northeast of Los Angeles decades earlier. "He designed it himself," Rosemary would celebrate, showing off Hank and the house at the same time. Hank was an aeronautics engineer; he built his lodge here, where he found consolation in crisp mountain air and rising peaks that reminded him of his distant youth in Austria. "The sun rises there." Hank would waggle a bony pointer at the glass door, across the canyon to the east. "And it advances all the way"—the finger semicircled in front of us—"to there." Hank would beam, pointing due west through another window, down the canyon, into the glare of the afternoon.

The house perched on a plateau just wide enough to hold it above the canyon, where it paid daily homage to the desert's extravagance with light. Below, the mountainside charged down two hundred feet, then scaled upward five hundred. Surrounding us like a mist, the dry, clean scent of pine baking in sunshine sprayed the air. A woodland of great pines, Coulter and Jeffrey, embraced the house, mixed with wild-branching live oaks, determined laurels, and ash-eating madrones. Once, a giant vulture, a California condor, gliding down a nine-foot wingspan, landed on the roof with a twenty-five-pound thud, its clomping claws gashing the roof like nails, at a time when the world population of condors numbered in the dozens. The Pine Mountain Club Fire Department had to go down to the house and climb up there to chase it off. Dropped on a thin spit of ridge in this high desert, Hank's remote mountain loft made a great asylum for a solitary artist or shelter for a laboring writer.

But it was not a home where Rosemary would entertain, as she used to so love to do when we were kids. My mother did not thrive in Pine Mountain Club, in the house that Hank built. Diabetes, fueled by the sugars in daily wine, destroyed her circulation and ability to walk; macular degeneration blackened her sight. In her eighties, her hearing dimmed to a faint ring. Mother's mind had been fading for a decade. When we took the wine away, finally, she seemed to recede and recede until there was hardly anything left of her.

Yet she had been quite a beauty and brightened so delightfully when she laughed, which was often in the good times, because she had a great sense of humor. Her brothers and sister in the Biritz clan loved to laugh, loved to play tricks on each other and giggle as they told the story ever after. Like the time Uncle Bernie convinced Uncle Sonny that sticking his arm out the passenger side of a 1960s Volkswagen Beetle would capsize the car. And the way they used to empty the filter tip on their cigarettes while they were sluicing martinis and stick them to the ceiling. If Aunt Margaret were visiting, they'd substitute Manhattans for the martinis.

They were all fun, the whole family. Uncle Jimmy convinced us little kids that the authorities were adding a day to the week—he called it Moonday—to balance out the number of days in the months. We were outside Linda's bedroom in the side yard, near the Bebb oak where I had buried five dollars in a small leather bag to find after a great hurricane or whirling tornado flattened our home. Its branches overhung the window box that poked out from Linda's room. "Oh yeah," Uncle Jimmy crooned at us, "just about the time I graduate, you guys will be getting an extra day every week." Uncle Jimmy was Grammy's surprise; he was only a few years older than Linda, Grammy's first grandchild. Jimmy was in high school. The big question was whether Moonday would be a school day or a weekend. Uncle Jimmy's friend on the inside heard they were leaning toward a school day. "If they don't make it a school day, they're going to add another month of school in the summer instead," he said, grinning cruelly. I nagged my mother for a week to find out.

But alcoholism is not all in fun. Being addicted is itself an agony of desperation and shame. The appalling impact on other people, particularly children, deepens the drinker's humiliation. Decent people descend into devastation. My parents drank like addicts and kept drowning to their predictable end. In AA, where I took refuge when I quit drinking in 1983, they used to tell me that alcohol, for ones such as we, would lead to illness, insanity, or death. We watched it lead to Daddy's early death in 1986. We missed its effects on Mom. One year, my stepdad called an ambulance for my mother twelve times. Somehow, we managed not to notice that wine was the cause of these mysterious falls and injuries.

In April, after Hank's death, Elizabeth moves in to care for Mom's basic needs. I could never have done that. Elizabeth loves dogs and other living things, but it's hard for me to understand how our younger sister, whom I still call Bethy, is willing to put this much attention and care into Mom. Mommy did not care for Elizabeth in her teen years. When Mom left Dad for Hank, she also left teenage Bethy homeless. Hank's children remained with their mother. Since Hank did not want children in his new home with Mom—an early clue into family dynamics that lasted beyond the grave—Bethy was out on her own. Daddy sank further into helplessness when Mom left; Bethy found a home with a high school friend. These many years later, when Mom is incompetent from dementia, Hank's will leaves their ragged estate to his eldest son, Larry, with instructions to care for Hank's youngest son. Elizabeth is not mentioned, yet she was the one who was abandoned as a child, and who is here to feed, clean, bathe, read to, and laugh with Mother to the end. Thus are we.

There is very little left of Mom in the three months she survives Hank. Her little body holds tender bones together with a few lingering, determined muscles that push her walker down her path to the bathroom every few hours. The walk is slow. One of us goes with her, following or leading the walker, through the doorways, turning on extra lights as we go. "Can't we turn on the lights?" she begs as we trudge. She can see only strong contrasts. She looks for spots of light as beacons on the dark passage. We are often too late for bowel movements, and this inevitably leads to a gentle but challenging cleanup. These terribly difficult, private moments leave one, as Linda will say later, little dignity. Mom insists that she do most of this for herself; the last bits of "what it is like to be Rosemary" remain obstinate. True to her own parenting commands, she washes her hands after every bathroom visit. At eighty-nine, she still insists on getting her hair and nails done, but after Hank's death her decline makes doing so wildly impractical. Elizabeth starts doing Mom's nails for her.

This is when Linda and I have the Big Fight. Linda and her husband, Rick, spend most of April searching for a residential care facility for Mom in Los Angeles, where Elizabeth and Linda can see her easily. Finally Linda finds a comfortable, homey facility nearby that will work with Mom's financial circumstances. She arranges for Mom to move in on a Wednesday. But nobody tells Mom! I feel strongly that Mom has to be informed and give consent, but Linda has a different view of how to care for Mommy with this dementia. I suspect she thinks it best to move Mom, get her comfortable, help her form new habits, and let her adjust, without forewarning and pre-upsetting her.

Anyway, she wants me out of it. She tells me my energy is too disruptive, that I am "frantic and constantly creating narrative, and endlessly self-centered." What does that even mean, "constantly creating narrative"? It means I talk too much. I am furious. (I do not know that a tumor is growing in Linda's abdomen and her doctor is keeping an eye on it.) Not only is she insulting me and discounting my input, but she also wants me out of the way. My image of three sisters working together with love is shattered. Something in me just goes hard and disconnects. I want Linda out of my life. But at the moment we have to focus on Mom.

I still insist we tell Mom that we are moving her. I have just forgotten she has no memory. On the Saturday morning before the planned move, I call. With a hearing-assistance telephone pressed against her left ear, she can hear me.

"Mom, we've been looking for a place where you could live closer to Linda and Beth. You could see them all the time. What would you think of that?"

"Leave my home? You want me to leave me home?"

"I know that sounds scary. I know. But we need to take care of you; you need daily help. We have to figure it out. If you're down there, they can get to you and we can get care for you."

"I can't I can't I am hanging up now." And she is gone; the phone drops. Someone hangs it up moments later.

Well, it's done, I think. *We've told her, and now we work it out and get her to go.*

In a few minutes, I get a text from Bethy: "What did you say to her? She's crying and says she won't leave her home." And then: "She's really upset. I'm going to get her some food and put on the TV and try to calm her down."

And then Mom forgets.

Elizabeth tells her again. And she forgets. Moving day is just a few days out. Bethy gives up telling Mom, unwilling to keep seeing her desperate and weepy reaction. Linda thinks we should go ahead with moving her, even though Mom never agreed. She's mad at me for telling Mom and getting things off track in the first place, and she tells me off. She begs me to back out of it and let her deal with Mom alone. I've never felt so discarded in my life, but a light starts to go on. I've been living in the dark about a lot of things.

When Wednesday comes and it is the moment to act, Bethy says no, she can't force Mom out the door. And the three of us just give up.

I tell Linda never to talk to me again, to just leave me alone.

Our younger stepbrother, Lenny, moves in to care for the house. I explain to Mom that the older son, Larry, is the executor of her property but that he is executing only in Mom's interest, with our support. Even in her confusion, she is oddly nervous about Larry's having control of the finances. Later, after she dies and I read the will, I understand why she has reservations about the arrangement. Larry already owns the house. Hank had declared Mom incompetent before he died.

Mom's strokes put her health in a terminal category that enables us to get her on hospice. Heaven-sent hospice nurses come to the house several times a week. Linda drives in for a day, or I come into town periodically, to relieve Elizabeth.

Linda also does the supply runs and helps manage the challenges of doctor visits. Doctor visits—good lord. Getting Mom dressed warmly enough in gentle clothing that will not hurt her skin. Getting food and pills allocated and packed. Getting out the door, getting down the steps, getting into the car. Hurrying her, too late, to a bathroom at the hospital. Cleaning up. Mommy enduring with patience, putting one foot in front of the other, pushing the walker one step at a time down hospital linoleum. Linda transports her through all this—the doctors, the tests, the consultations. We three daughters have this same tenacity. We will pull the whole train up the mountain by ourselves with our teeth if no one is going to help.

When I visit, we eat at the round dining table sandwiched between the living room couch and the half wall bordering Hank's library. This table hosted all Mom and Hank's meals, the plates set on red faux-leather placemats next to black cloth napkins gathered in wooden napkin rings. She and Hank were in a regular dietary rhythm for years to accommodate their various medications. Hank would place little piles of pills under the eaves of the plates. With Mom in decline, we find the frequent ritual of having a snack or small meal at this table a welcome distraction and comfort. We get Mom over to eat three times a day, even if just a snack of peanut butter with apple, dishing out pills at each meal. Sometimes after she eats she sits in her dining chair while Elizabeth or I brush her hair, which by then falls straight and nearly to her shoulders. As her hair grows longer, gentle brushing gives her periods of deep rest.

When Elizabeth and I are together at Mom's for more than a few hours, we start to irritate each other. A painful tension exists between us, but I cannot discern what it is about. An outsider would see two women struggling to maintain patience and self-control under great strain. It seems like there are resentments hanging in the air. Am I harboring something? Did I do something? My mind is too foggy with everything going on for me to see clearly. Sometimes whatever I do seems to cause upset or drive Bethy out of the room. Other moments flow. We get by and get through it. We aren't able to give each other much comfort. My mind is in a kind of haze state, my movements plodding. When you go into the house of the dying, you go into an alternate dimension, with a slow, quiet quality of life, your attention just here. Nothing much happens, but it is exhausting.

I sleep on the couch in the living room, a small capsule of space squeezed between the bedroom and the dining table. Elizabeth sleeps in the bedroom with Mom, and Lenny sleeps on the foldout in Hank's den. The den fills nearly half of the house. The other half—the half we girls were all in—contains the master bedroom, living room, dining area, bathrooms, and kitchenette. Designing his dream home, Hank left out Mother's needs entirely, but she went along with it. His den has floor-to-ceiling windows looking out on a vast California high-desert canyon. Mom has a desk in the bedroom corner. "Mom, are you sure you don't want a reading chair or something out in the den?" "No, this is fine." Mom needed family. Mom needed friends, a social life, a fabric of life to belong to. A chair in Hank's den, though not offered, would not have helped. Years went by. Mom faded.

Hank's den comprises seven six-by-ten-foot bookshelves, jutting out from the wall like teeth on a comb, each filled with volumes, and a six-by-three-foot corner desk. This library, where he explored phys-ical science (particularly Einstein) and mathematics (particularly

Mandelbrot) presented his imagined orderly, rule-bound, and engineerable world of the mid-twentieth century. The collection also includes histories, Arthur Conan Doyle, all of Bertrand Russell and Einstein, some biographies. It weighs tons, having anchored Hank and Mom in this wilderness. Hank said he could never move without his bookshelves.

Along the carpet path my mother treads every few hours from the couch or dining table, through the bedroom to the bathroom, a series of brown stains tears at my self-possession. How has my glamorous mother come to this terribly fragile state? I get on all fours and scrub those marks with kitchen cleanser and a few tears, something with bleach, something to take out the discoloration and the memories and the pain, fading the knees of the light gray stretch jeans that my partner, Jill, gave me for Christmas.

It's my sixty-fifth birthday this year, in early June. A couple weeks before Mom dies, I am at her place, giving Beth a little break. Once, we order out—good, hot Mexican food. Once, Elizabeth cooks. Twice, we have microwaved frozen dinners. I forget what we do for dinner this evening. Elizabeth, and you must try to picture this, is single-handedly providing minute-by-minute care, including all the things I haven't mentioned: buying, preparing, and serving food; cleaning up; dressing Mom; doing laundry; dealing with hospice and showers; leading regular bathroom marches; dosing medicines two or three times a day; tracking status; and calling for help when needed. She is walking the final path step by step. But do you know what else that girl does? She remembers my birthday, and she gets us an ice cream cake roll with a candle in it.

In the midst of that intensity—where the outside world has no impact on the central drama playing out in the few hundred square feet holding we three girls—Elizabeth emerges from the kitchenette singing "Happy Birthday," cake with flaming candle aloft. Then Mom, who barely understands I am there, lifts her face to the sound of Bethy's voice and joins the song—"Happy birthday, dear Rikki, happy birthday to you"—in her kind voice, her comforting-mother voice, though thin and dying. I feel loved. I feel connected, I know my mother feels connected and feels loved and it matters, and that can happen even though we are Demented and Bewildered. Bethy gives me the bestest-ever birthday present: my mom's love for one more moment, before she leaves us forever.

I watch for any ways to give Mom some relief or some experience of comfort or pleasure. I bring homegrown roses for her to smell. I prepare homemade soup with roasted potatoes from the garden that Mom helped plant a few years earlier. I read the beginning of Chapter 5 of *The Red Tent*, a rhythmically told tale of desert women and the peaceful rituals of their steady lives. Each day I read the beginning of the same chapter. Each day, it is new to Mom. After a few days, several images stick with her. She knows what's coming: "Isn't there a girl with her?" she says.

I'm not ashamed that I often wish for Mom to die quickly and with as little pain as possible, within a few months of Hank's death. We are blessed that it turns out that way. I cannot understand how this fate overran her. And yet *do* I know? And do I want to run from knowing?

FINDING PATTERNS
Santa Cruz Mountains
August 2016

I know that much of Mom's decline she did to herself. It sounds bitterly harsh, but I am trying to face up to our harmful family patterns. I don't mean simply that she brought her demise on herself through destructive drinking, although that is true. She did sign on to the party life with my father, who had a wild streak of savage self-hatred that might erupt on her at any time. Dad had demons, and scotch, and money, and a successful Chicago advertising firm that specialized in comedic spots. He drank to work; they drank after work; he drank to calm down; she drank to recover from his verbal violence and abuse. He wrote funny ads and acted out; she raised three kids, ran the household, and blamed him for the loneliness and confusion that often flooded her. It was Mom's conscious adult choices that put her there. But other, invisible forces locked them together in an ongoing, strangled drama.

What I mean is that each of us undermines our own life efforts in our own unique way. We bring it on ourselves, unconscious though we may be. My mother slowly gave her power away until she had none. Many women in her generation lived in the world through the men they married. But my mom married self-seekers who let her fade while she waited to be seen and validated. She let the unconscious victim in her be victimized.

Learning from my mother, I see that I also unwittingly complicate situations for myself and sabotage my efforts with unconscious patterns. Self-pity made my Nokia experience harder for me without my realizing it or being able to stop myself. I've watched myself seem to strive for a goal, yet the way I react to obstacles ensures I will give up or fail. A deep-seated sense of being life's victim can lead me to make choices and take actions that unconsciously re-create victim-y situations without my ever knowing about it. This sort of mysterious impulse can create insidious conditions in real life. Sometimes you set up recurring painful relationship dynamics that repeatedly show you how it felt, deep inside unconscious you, when some pattern originally formed. I get my old childish feelings activated too easily and let them throw me for a loop. That kind of thing can leave you confused and frustrated if you don't understand how the pattern works in you.

Or take intimacy. I feel vaguely ill at ease if basic communication flow is blocked. It doesn't take much for me to notice, and it makes me uncomfortable. I try to pull you closer. But intimacy actually makes me feel threatened, even consumed, so I also push you away, unconsciously creating some distance. Conflicting compulsions take hold of neurological and hormonal processes when one of these patterns is at work. You work against yourself.

You don't know why, but you keep undermining certain things, even though you're doing everything right. You have the same fight over and over with your disgruntled partner. You get in the same situation at work. I suspect that I sabotaged my career each time I moved toward deeper career satisfaction. I just wish I'd known how unconscious aversions manipulated me at earlier choice points. Did I worm my way out of great opportunities? Was I able to take my best shots? How about now, in retirement?

One of the worst scenarios is what I call the memento complex, after the wife in the 2001 movie *Memento*. The lead male has lost the ability to form new memories. To shock him out of this condition, his wife asks him for her diabetes medication every hour, knowing he should recall having done the previous injections, knowing the overdose will kill her. He kills her; she lets him—hoping against hope that he will suddenly realize what is going on and save her. She gives her life away for that hope. Giving yourself up while hoping someone will see you and value you more than you do yourself is the memento complex.

My mom became like this. She neglected herself and surrendered her power while waiting to be seen, loved, saved, or rescued. Although we could see her, we could not rescue her. She knew; she saw it in herself. I learned it from her. She used to catch me just as I was giving something away, a jacket or my time: "Don't give yourself away so easily, Rikki." Takes one to know one. A favorite song of my mother's, which seemed gay and lighthearted at the time, now echoes with foreboding: "Que Sera, Sera." Whatever will be, will be. As if you have no agency, as if you are hardly here.

She couldn't save me from myself—I had to learn from consequences—and I couldn't do her work for her. Everyone has to work out his or her own salvation. Taking on the role of codependent martyr to my father's drunken abuse, my mother slowly developed into a helpless victim. You don't even realize it's happening. Even when she left my father, she turned to another self-absorbed intellectual who couldn't see her. In midlife, Rosemary eluded my father's shadow to settle down in Henry's dark sanctuary.

Hank was born in Graz, Austria. Graz was the first Austrian city from which the Nazis expelled the entire Jewish population—several thousand citizens. Not all of his family made it out. He and his parents escaped in 1938 by train and then by ship out of Italy. They steamed down the Adriatic from Trieste into the Mediterranean, out through the narrow Strait of Gibraltar, and into the Atlantic. He drew the route on the map in my world atlas for me. Every year, he acknowledged his family's date of arrival in New York. Hank was thirteen. When I was thirteen, I read most of *The Diary of Anne Frank*. It frightened me, so I simply stopped reading it. It's hard for me to believe what Hank went through.

In 2000, the residents of Graz dedicated a small synagogue built on the site where the large-domed nineteenth-century temple was destroyed on Kristallnacht in 1938. Some burned, blackened stones, preserved from the original foundation, form a small memorial wall behind the temple. Surviving former students from around the world were invited. Hank and Mom made the journey with Linda and Rick, who, also Jewish, lost family in Europe as well. The four even made a pilgrimage to the family apartment where Hank lived until his family's forced expulsion. Hank soared to hero status in my mind for going. It took a lot of guts on my mother's part, too. But he remained an isolated and self-absorbed man. How could he not?

"Henry," she would say, "you need a new pair of shoes," every time she needed shoes. She just couldn't bring herself to demand more love and attention than the narcissists around her offered. Almost incidentally, without knowing it, she diminished herself until there was scarcely anything left but a wisp of love when she died. It was heartbreaking to watch over the last years.

Many of my unconscious patterns seem to be unwitting variations on my parents' themes. I have my father's arrogance, with its condescending, sarcastic voice. More dangerous, I think I have his demons, his self-hatred and anger. I have my mother's timidity, with its tendency to surrender personal power, and its demon: resentment of power.

My patterns can be destructive and vicious. They have undermined important efforts of mine in career and family. The remorseless way they play out in me is humbling. But, as the legend says about the Buddha, I've discovered that there is a way out. The good news is, patterns can be dislodged and released. I've been rooting them out intentionally using tools from AA, yoga, and American Zen. The bad news is, these methods can take time: I've been doing this for thirty-five years.

I vowed to root out my character-destructive tendencies that are reminiscent of my mother's, but not her kindness. I covet that. "Your mom is the sweetest thing," we heard from friends old and new. "Good listening makes a good friend." Rosemary listened when people spoke; she attended. This is my most precious skill, for which I rarely praised or thanked my mother. But it is a scarce gift. How many people do you know who look you in the eyes while you are speaking and don't let their mind fill with what they have to say about it? It's a natural capacity my sisters and I have.

I'd like very much to use it to listen to Linda and to myself. But there's a lot going on right now. My equilibrium is thrown way off. My mother has just died, and my big sister is facing death or worse, and we haven't spoken to each other for months. I feel confused and disoriented. It's like standing in slashing strips of rain—everything seems sort of obscured and hard to think about. When I listen, I just hear wailing. Still, though I can't say how, I am certain I will be very strong and stand up for my sister and find ways to be present for her. I will listen and I will be kind and Mommy will be proud of us.

I want to tap authentic trust, cheerful spirits, and some kind of openness to let things take their natural course. Relaxing is always a last-ditch effort for me. If I set the intention, at least, to relax into my natural, whole self, perhaps I will find it is already at peace.

That's what I need: a place to stand where I feel at peace. Right now I feel like I am flying through space without any ground. Linda needs a *stem cell transplant*. There is an active and growing tumor that will *kill* her. The words make no sense.

GRAPPLING

HIGH ASPIRATIONS
Santa Cruz Mountains
August 2016

Once you are at wits' end, if you don't get a grip on it, things can keep slipping. Daddy's drinking and depression drove Mommy to her wits' end. Mommy's family did not help her deal with the challenges Dick posed.

"You married him; you have to stick with him," her brother said.

"That's marriage. You take care of him, and he'll drink less," her mother said.

But it wasn't just marriage. It was alcohol addiction, and it wasn't going to change. This was the initial collapse of spirit for Mom. This is the way family addiction operates. Mom gave in to her powerlessness in the situation, instead of finding some other possibility. The future collapses just happened. It's harder to stop something once it's running downhill.

I learned that pattern.

But I don't think Linda did. The inside of her head is different from mine; her emotions work differently. The kind of support I might want is not a good guide to what Linda might want. We cope in our own ways.

I know my parents ridiculed her, as they did me. My father called her names, like Flibbertigibbet, whatever that means, and Eeyore, from *Winnie-the-Pooh*. Why did they have to say it with sarcasm, with derision? Drinking made them nasty, but it didn't help us that sarcastic and insulting humor was popular at the time. Lenny Bruce was my father's idol. Don Rickles was a popular put-down artist. Insults were a matter of wit; the target should be able to take it. But I didn't like them teasing her. She was my hero. I don't know how it affected her. I never thought to ask. I was busy juggling my own collapse, trying to find banisters. While I became super-sensitive, I suspect Linda wrapped a cool protective cloak around her fragile child's shoulders.

I don't know how she processed these family dynamics in her young life. Each of us has so much that is private, deeply personal, hidden in the crevices. I marvel that anyone can ever connect with another person. I want to be intimate with Linda and Rick, but intimacy is so risky. Every approach carries the risk of rejection, even ridicule. From childhood you have the scars to show it. How do you rise beyond that to trust an intimacy with another person? You have to trust that person to have your best interests at heart. At heart, though, is a dark and mysterious place—deep, fickle, hidden. How does anyone even know what is in his or her own heart? Perhaps only with mindfulness after a long life.

Home in the Santa Cruz Mountains, I write in a journal for a while, unpacking the material that just came in the course of the day, clearing some space to feel what I am feeling. I watch while thoughts and emotions move through my mind. Here is a tedious, repetitive review of a conversation with my neighbor. Then there's envy of my friend with plenty of money. Here's unanchored self-blame that's a residue of feeling responsible for other people's lives. I worry whether I did enough for Linda and Rick. The will to dominate comes up while playing Words With Friends. Competitiveness spikes when talking with a successful colleague. So many ways the mind moves that I rather regret. It seems such a waste of time.

Around 5:30 p.m., I feed our American Staffordshire terrier mix, Zoey, and take out the stuff I'm making for dinner. I prep the veggies for a stir-fry: asparagus, carrots, mushrooms, broccoli. Jill comes home around 7:00 p.m. Her long, straight brown hair is usually tied back behind her neck, bangs loose at the front and sides. Tonight there is more loose than usual, perhaps a sign of traffic troubles. She has a cute, round, elfin face that simply delights you when she's laughing, but when she's angry, her scowl can be frightening. I'm scanning her face, half hidden behind her Maui Jims, when a smile breaks out. "Hi, baby!" she calls out. All is good. I hear someone exhaling. It's me. Jill unloads her stuff and sets the table for dinner.

Although California law allows us to get married, we are actually registered domestic partners or, as we affectionately call ourselves, DOMPAs. We got together when my daughter was in tenth grade. She was homeschooling that year, an arrangement we worked out with the homeschool supervisor at her high school. She had to follow the regular curriculum. She and I studied the social movements and wars of the twentieth century, second-year algebra, and literature. I was sure I understood the algebra, but my word problems did not come out right; I was not much help to her there. When she got to literature about wars, I couldn't read along. Anne Frank and Elie Wiesel demanded too much of me emotionally. I was sorry my little baby had to learn about this part of humanity. My little baby who, a few years earlier in grade school, found out that children in our world today are kept and traded as slaves for labor and sex, and then started a group she called the Eye Club to raise awareness in our town. "We must keep our eye on the world," she told me.

Romance with a woman was all new to Jill, but not to me. I came out in 1978, to help defeat the so-called Briggs Initiative in California, which would have made it illegal for suspected gay men and lesbians to teach in public schools. As happened so often in the '70s, I was politically motivated by music. At a women's concert in Berkeley, singer Holly Near asked us all to "come out" to our friends and neighbors, showing them that the gay person they knew was fit to teach children. Terrified but committed, I came out to friends, family, and coworkers. No one was surprised. No one rejected or abandoned me. The penny dropped for all of us. The Briggs Initiative failed—a victory for us. I never questioned my gayness again, but I instinctively hid my sexuality and my alcoholism from new acquaintances even after that.

Jill took a different route. She got married after beginning her professional career at IBM. Eventually she left that marriage. When we were dating I would tease her, saying, "I'm a lesbian, but my girlfriend isn't." She has been incredibly patient with me since Linda's email. In fact, she's been encouraging and supportive all these months since my mother's illness, which took up so much of my time and attention.

We eat our dinner while watching the news and a TV drama. I'm only half here. I'm unsettled about the risks facing Linda. She's learned that she needs butt-kicking chemotherapy right away to keep the tumor from compromising her organ function and bringing death within months. But the lymphoma doctors know they can't kill this tumor; they can only beat it back, in hopes that the stem cell transplant, at the right moment, will, if everything goes perfectly, eventually bring about tumor destruction. I can't seem to grok that she could actually die and then not be here with our family anymore. It's too much to take onboard tonight. Underneath all those thoughts, I tune my attention to a quiet place, like a womb, in the center of my chest, and breathe. When we trundle off to bed, I can't remember what show we just watched.

I awaken with a dark-of-night convulsion of fear that I've ruined something. I simply don't know what it is yet.

I just want her to live. Since the Big Fight, I've understood that my energy can be challenging for Linda, especially under chemo. I'll provide better support if my drama doesn't drown out either of us. I can keep my energy quiet and get myself aligned with the intention of supporting her through this. That will enable me to read situations better and avoid creating upset. *There's just too much of me, I think, and not enough room for us both. Let's make more room for Linda right now.* (Later, I will have to straighten out my bent tendency to deal myself out of every hand.)

"I thought I was ready to die, but I don't want to," Linda tells me. I picture her knitting while talking into her headset. Her fingers push the twine along a needle. "I want to go to dance class and travel to Lake Tahoe with my book club." Like a match igniting a pile of dry kindling, that burns my heart. "Instead, I'm going to start a six-month cycle of chemo." It will keep her isolated, indoors at home, and vulnerable the whole time.

My best friend, Terri, when she was dying, wrote that she just wanted to sort her sock drawer. Simple acts that you can do when you're alive. The thought makes my chest tighten and throat close for Linda and for myself and all vulnerable beings. Tenderness for that simple longing everyone has: to be, not to end, yet. To see what's next.

I know somehow I have to be present with Linda through this ordeal. We are childhood co-survivors. Whether she knows how much she needs me or not, I am showing up. Like the song says, I'll be with her when the deal goes down.

So if my arrogance or self-centeredness or jabbertalk makes me annoying, I will simply dial it all back. I'll get my whole self centered on a single aspiration. All fibers aligned, concentrating on a single goal.

An aspiration had grown in me over the years as I wrestled with my ambitions and struggled with my life questions. As an inherently empathic person, I feel the pain of others without seeking to. My imagination takes me into their shoes uninvited. It will fill up with concern, or pity, or sadness for another's plight. In Buddhist circles, I heard an aspiration that helped me navigate the sorrows I encounter without losing my equilibrium: "May I be free of suffering. May all beings be free of suffering." These words help me deal with the heaviness of the feelings I absorb when I encounter pain, and they cheer me. As I work with my own mind and its confusion, I've begun to believe all beings *can* find some freedom. Getting aligned with the quest for that freedom helps me get a fresh perspective on my own confusion. I've begun to *feel* the aspiration to awaken and help free all beings.

I often make this aspiration for individuals: "May so-and-so be free of suffering." But, frankly, I don't like the focus on suffering. An article in *Lion's Roar* magazine turned me on to a variation I do like: "May all beings feel the joy of their own hearts beating in their own chests." It has an uplifting feel that spontaneously rouses my spirits. Whether we realize it or not, our raised spirits, clear minds, and happy energy enliven other people. Plus, you can say to your big sister, "My prayer for you is this: may you feel the joy of your own heart beating in your own chest." It sounds a lot better than "May you be free from suffering."

In this situation, the aspiration that comes to me is to be a loving presence for Linda through thick and thin and to not be annoying. "May I be a loving presence and not annoying," I hum.

The prayer "May I not be annoying" is pretty uninspiring and too self-deprecating, but it is sincere. Sincerity is like willingness; it has a purity that draws the best from the depths, even when your thinking is a little off. I really, really do not want to irritate Rick or Linda while I am supporting them. If it means repressing my personality, I'm down with that. The dangerous part for me is thinking that my annoying parts are actually annoying—like, actually bad or broken according to some universal laws. That is incorrect thinking. That is the kind of ignorance or delusion that causes suffering. My annoying behaviors are just behaviors that someone is reacting to. It doesn't mean there is something wrong with me.

For myself I make a vow: "I vow to awaken for the sake of all beings. I vow not to abandon myself and to continue until I befriend myself completely. May I feel the joy of my own heart beating in my own chest." I don't see yet the many ways I abandon myself. But my vow has surely set me on a good trajectory.

I don't know what it means to awaken, but I am interested. Part of it seems to involve locating unconscious patterns and loosening their control. Once I have stopped being fooled by an unconscious pattern, I see it working and it loses its power. Spontaneously, understanding and compassion for myself arise right there. Whatever I need seems to be there if I can just loosen the strangling grip of the delusion. There's real freedom in making friends with myself.

My aspirations fuel this clear intention: Deliver an abundance of potent, healthy stem cells that will protect Linda's health, will attack any cancer cells, and won't attack Linda's body cells. My meditation will help spruce up the energetic health of the environment those cells grow in. And my Muay Thai kickboxing will sharpen all the cells in my body, tuning them to high performance.

GRAPPLING WITH OUR MINDS
Santa Cruz Mountains
August 2016

To really thrive, I've had to grapple with the unconscious habits of my own mind. Most of us have not thought about this concept. Our minds drive us hither and yon. Thoughts and feelings arise unbidden; unconscious pressures, memories, and resentments nag us; envies and worries press upon us. But that ephemeral quality of mind does not have to toss your inner life around. The quality of your inner life depends on how you grapple with your own mind.

I say this with the conviction of the nearly damned. I had to learn to grapple with my mind because of my alcohol addiction. I had to listen and get my defenses to soften so I could tell myself what was behind the confusion and pain my mind presented to me uninvited. Learning to relax and open my own mind took a long time. You are doing it from the inside with your own weird thoughts, so it gets to be kind of a whirligig project.

My relationship with my mind began with a baggie stuffed with Maui Wowie that Kim Jordan and I acquired from Ranch Trent, up the street, for ten bucks, in fall 1966. We were going to smoke it and go to the Friday-night varsity game at Birmingham High School in Van Nuys, California.

Fall 1966

Kim drove over after dinner, and we went quietly up to my room. I lit a stick of incense to hide the scent and stuck it in the incense holder on my dresser, on top of the *Rubber Soul* album cover. I grabbed a shoebox lid, and Kim emptied the baggie into it. Holding the lid at an angle, I raked my fingers through the stash, filtering out stems and breaking up clumps. We got a pretty clean pile of weed. Kim had rolling paper. I washed the sticky residue off my fingers while she tried to roll a joint. Her first try left a shredded, wet glob of paper wrapped helplessly around a grassy mess. Next time we glued two papers together, and she rolled the paper around a pencil to get a curl in it before she loaded in our lumpy weed. Rolling it gently back and forth between her fingertips, she made a tube packed with our stash, licked the edge, and sealed it. She twisted the ends and held up joint number one. "Voilà!" The third try went more smoothly, but the Wowie stick was just as lumpy.

We both already smoked cigarettes and knew how to inhale. I was fifteen; Kim was sixteen and had a car for the night; she had to be home by 10:00 p.m. We lit up those two fat doobies, chunky with shredded leaf. We smoked them down, tapping the ember to keep a steady burn on the unevenly packed weed. Neither of us had thought to acquire a roach clip, but I found a bobby pin in the bath-room drawer and we used that. Slowly, an odd, glowing sensation infused me; an intense self-consciousness bloomed, and I began to laugh. Kimmy was staring at her shoe, fascinated. "You never notice how beautiful shoes really are," she said happily.

Stumbling down the front stairs, we sang the lyrics to "Like a Rolling Stone" and giggled our way into the kitchen. We grabbed some bags of chips. My mom caught us in the kitchen, talking rapidly and laughing. "You girls have a good time tonight!" She smiled. "Will do, Mrs. West," Kimmy chirped. My mom was not looking for trouble. *Happy girls are good enough girls*, she would think. "Go, have fun," Mom said. I had turned on. I would tune in. I would question authority. I would question everything. I started following Maharishi Mahesh Yogi, the Beatles' guru. It really did not take long to discover that the principal thing stopping me, strangling me, was me. I did not yet understand how to work with myself, how to work with the tendencies and patterns in my mind. But something was stimulated. In 1967, I gave up the acid and the pot. A few years later I read *Be Here Now*.

After a rocky beginning, my relationship with my mind seemed on track. There were just a couple of unconscious mental patterns that could give me a bit of trouble. For example, I did begin to drink a lot in college. And by the time I was in graduate school in the late 1970s, I was a character at the daytime bar across the street from my part-time job. Happy hour was all the rage in those days. I passed out almost every night, not always in a familiar bed. Drinking came easily, like bullets sliding into a chamber. My drinking was naturally destructive. I blacked out, hid bottles, stole from anyone, lied to friends, cheated on lovers. It's a tale for another time, and one that has been told by millions of now-sober comrades. There was nothing individually interesting about my drinking. Long story short, booze and self-criticism beat me to pieces. I had no relationship with my mind. Really there were just a lot of patterns running, in which I was a passive dupe. I had no game plan, nobody home to learn the game. You are always recovering, planning, or drinking, with no cycles free to attend to yourself. You don't realize it, though—you convince yourself that you're just having a good time.

And I had secretly implanted the memento complex. I had buried the best part of me, the most creative and vulnerable, the kernel, where she would never be shamed and would wait futilely for someone else to validate her. That led to a series of choices that left me out of the equation. I thought I was pursuing my interests, but I was also profoundly neglecting myself, waiting for someone to come consider me and authenticate me. I hid my talents while trying to accomplish goals you valued, so you would validate me. I denied myself while promoting you, hoping you would value me for that. It was a failure of boundaries. It was a failure of self. I had failed to experience the source of power in my life coming from within me. I was waiting for someone else to fuel my rocket. I had trapped myself unknowingly to protect myself.

It seems my psyche did this on its own, without asking permission. Clues to this twist were in the kinds of suffering this cognitive strategy created for me. Only much later would I discover various ways in which I wrote myself out of the story, and how that did not work out well. How I would give away my time, energy, and resources to others in acts of what they call idiot compassion. You don't help anyone, really; you just give away your energy to calm your anxieties.

In Muay Thai kickboxing, you have a situation to grapple with that is very much like grappling with your mind. You step into the ring with nothing but yourself—no weapon, no phone, no team of people to back you up. You can't bring your lawyer or your money. The car you drive is out in the parking lot, where it can do you no good. You have your shin guards, mouth guard, and boxing gloves. The person staring at you is waiting for the bell to ring so they can legally walk over to you and hit and kick you as much possible. When the bell rings, it's chaos! You forget to take a good stance because your attention has flown over there to the adversary. Suddenly, a very long jab is hitting your head, and you stand there stupidly before getting your hands up and remembering you have feet. Move! But you've sidestepped into a body kick, even worse. Blows from everywhere leave you backing into a corner, with no way out.

In the ring, the first thing you have to do is get your stance. Everything before that is just flailing helplessly, dominated by the blows from your sparring partner.

The stance in Muay Thai is different from that in boxing. In boxing you take a bladed stance, turning your side to the opponent and tucking in behind your lead shoulder. This is great if the only incoming strikes are from fists, but Muay Thai is the Art of Eight Limbs. You have legal strikes coming in from knees, shins, and elbows. It's much more chaotic and like real life in that way. You get into a stance that allows you to defend any of these strikes from a neutral position. You return to neutral after every sequence of moves. You square your hips to your opponent and drop your rear leg back about a shoulder's width, and you stand tall. Knees are flexed but not bent like in boxing. You can deal with everything from here. Then you learn to move and strike in clever ways that let you return to neutral, like landing a hook to the body when you recenter after a hard, straight right.

Once you get a stance, you can start to see what is happening in the ring. *Where is that strike coming from? How did I miss when I threw that teep? Why am I getting kicked?* It takes a while to see the moves, the sequence, and then the rhythm. It's just the same in grappling with my mind. I have to get a stance with some distance from the emotion or pattern that is taking over my sparring session. A witness stance lets me get in a position where I can view what is arising without getting swept away by it. Sitting, I get quiet and find my witness stance; I breathe and center. I observe the rising of tension in my chest; maybe the sensation feels "orange" and enclosing, like strangling. I trace the emotion that comes with it, like sadness or regret or rage or confusion. Then I let all that be and watch it slow down so I can start to deal with it.

For the incoming jab, once you can see what's happening, you have many options. Lean back, slip to the side, or step away. Parry or catch. Or take the jab, step in, and deliver two clean uppercuts. You just need the presence of mind to execute. Presence of mind is the key. That can come only from practice and understanding. You have to understand what you're doing and practice it repeatedly so your mind learns to choose that pattern, rather than the unconscious panic of its past.

In grappling with the mind, you have to slow things down until you can see what's happening. You need the presence of mind to sort things out. I had to quit drinking so I could begin to see what was happening in me. I needed a lot of stabilization from the steps, the community, and the structure of the recovery process before I could see very much. Deep within my psyche, conflicting, self-negating fragments and impressions failed to cohere into a whole-enough self. Unconscious patterns ran various rackets that gave me a false sense of having my stuff together, but I didn't know what clothes I liked to wear. I didn't know how I liked to wear my hair. I lacked a healthy self-concept to sponsor my adult enterprise. I was a thirty-something-year-old software project manager who felt like a little boy, wanted to look like Bob Dylan, and tried to fit in with straight, left-brained, boomer-age technologists, all the while hiding from everyone the troublesome facts of being both alcoholic and lesbian.

I got to AA a couple of years after landing my first job post–graduate school, in 1981, and I was clean and sober by the time I was thirty-two. I struggled with the 12 Steps. I didn't want to admit I needed help. I didn't want to ask for help from a higher power. That felt shameful; only broken people need that. Now, as I write this book, I can't remember why I thought it was shameful to need help. I don't know why I thought I should know how to do life. Where would I have learned? The principles embodied in the 12 Steps reshaped my thinking and helped me get a persistent sense of stability. AA taught me a new way of relating to myself and the world. The steps showed me how to take responsibility for the impact of my life, no matter how much it bewildered me. People in the community showed me through their lives how you take responsibility for your impact and your future. They gave me a specific set of things I could do for myself to get help, to get insight, to get freedom from despair. AA put me on my own two feet.

I learned I never had to be alone again, although I would be lonely. I learned I never had to be done in by darkness or confusion or self-hatred, though these would rise up. I discovered I could relax, saying, "This too shall pass." Following the guidance in the Big Book, I wrote down my existing resentments one by one. I was lucky enough to see my part in the way they soured my mind, and to let go of my stories and insistence on being right. I made amends for ruined relationships and trails of arrogant neglect.

Doing the steps changes you in the same way that loss and grief carve new landscapes in your heart. These are not easy steps to walk. In AA, you need not walk them alone. In meetings around the world, in multiple languages, I found AA friends who knew what to say and how to listen. "Don't quit before the miracle," I often heard. So often, a solution will work itself out in time, but the agitated mind has to learn patience. "Do you want to be happy or right?" someone would ask pointedly.

"I want to be right! I would rather be right than happy!" was my first response. But then life beats you up until you are willing to let it go. For this experience, AA offers the slogan "Let go and let God." These days, I'd rather be happy than right. It turns out that being right is the booby prize.

The steps became the thing that I reach for in the dark to deal with the monsters that arise in my own mind. The eleventh step encouraged me to develop a habit of meditation, reflection, and prayer that serves me every day. That led me to yoga and Zen. There is always something in the 12 Steps that will help me when I get stuck. They are a complete guide for sparring in real life.

So it's with conviction that I say, if you are anything like me, we have to grapple with our minds. And you're probably a little like me. It's obvious if you are alcoholic, but everyone else has demons, too. They're just more subtle, or clever.

FINDING MY COMPOSURE

Santa Cruz Mountains
August 2016

I drop my bright yellow Adidas gym bag on the floor and root around in it, pushing boxing mitts to one end. I pull out mouth guard, kerchief, orange hand tape, and my blue ten-ounce gloves. The gym smells like sweat, and it's cold in here. One guy is jumping rope, and a woman is doing yoga stretches over by the bags. I leave my sweats on over my shorts and tank and pop the clear polyvinyl mold into my mouth. The red-checked kerchief gets threaded through the handle of my purple metal water bottle. I keep my water bottle near me all the time; it's not de rigueur during class to take water breaks, but I sip at each transition. I'm a senior citizen, and I give myself a special dispensation to drink a lot of water. There's a sticker on my bottle that proclaims BADASS! just in case anyone thinks water is for wimps.

I take the time to wrap my hands well. Jake told me to treat it like a ritual to prepare myself for the coming battle. I used to rush through it, embarrassed by the clumsiness of my technique. The wraps are fifteen feet long, and you wind them around your wrist and around each finger and thumb repeatedly. These protect your hands inside the gloves when you're hitting the bag or focus mitts as hard as you can. We have drills for speed, drills for technique, and drills for power. I've injured my hands during power drills; now I wrap carefully. Over the knuckles of my left hand, wrap five times. Set that pad on my knuckles, then wrap around the wrist, over between thumb and forefinger, then back around the wrist. Repeat between forefinger and middle and around the wrist. I give myself permission to take my own time. Get the tape flat. This is for me. This is how I find my composure. Sitting next to me on the floor are two fighters in red Muay Thai shorts with KOA written across the front, naming our gym. They are wrapping their hands with similar tapes.

Jake taught me about composure. He'd have me sprint a length of sidewalk and back at my absolute full-out best speed, maybe just fifty yards, and as I bent over, gasping and sucking, he'd sweep his hands together, then apart, like a conductor gathering the orchestra. "In through the nose . . ." The hands semicircled from under his nose, down and outward. "Out through the mouth . . ." The hands swept down from a blessing and into a prayer. "In through the nose. Out through the mouth. Regain your composure."

Composure? I thought, the first time. I was heaving; I was gasping; I was letting my upper body flop around and pump like a busted bellows. *Composure?* I gathered myself together and stood still while, carefully and steadily, I breathed through my nose. *Wow.* Clarity snapped like a camera's shutter. *That's something I could really use,* I thought. So I wrap my hands attentively.

I get out on the floor, grab a jump rope, check the clock, and start a three-minute set. I won't make it through without a few stumbles, but it's a great warm-up and helps with my core alignment. Core is key to kickboxing. It took me a long time to realize that. Just watch how a boxer's body moves, versus a runner's. Shoulder, waist, and hip move as a solid unit.

My lungs really start to pull at around two minutes, and my mind gets tense, so I count to distract it. One, two, three . . . up to eight. Then I start again. One, two, three . . . When the three-minute bell rings, I'm still going strong. I put away the jump rope, grab a pair of three-pound dumbbells, and start a three-minute shadowboxing set. My imaginary opponent starts out as my image in the mirror. I whip out a series of jabs that would crack her chin. Twisting quickly to the right to slip the imaginary incoming jab, I think, *Remember, weight balanced on your back foot*, in case a front kick is coming after the cross and I want to get my leg up to block. I can't get that front leg up if I put my weight on it when I twist right.

I keep my balance and throw up the block. Then pivot, jab-jab, cross, hook-hook. Move. Pivot. Keep moving, throwing punches with the weights for three minutes. This is a great time to fantasize, or what in sports psychology they call *visualize*. I can't ever quite picture myself hitting a real person, though. I suppose that could hurt my long-term fighting prospects.

Going at my own pace, I avoid doing kicks while I'm holding the weights. No need to invite injuries.

Next I do three minutes of shadowboxing without weights. Now I throw it all in: full roundhouse kicks to head and body; teeps to the belly and leg; all the hand strikes, head and body. Jab-cross to the head, cross to the body. Jab-jab, cross, uppercut-uppercut. Bah, bah, tap-tap, boom. Getting into a rhythm, I picture myself as an easy, fluid kickboxer deflecting punches and landing devastating head strikes. I think, *Footwork*, and I start to move around more, as if I were really avoiding an opponent while staying close enough in to strike. I think, *Combos*, and I throw a two-one-two left leg kick, then a one-two-one right body kick. The three minutes pass like spilled water. I'm working up a good sweat.

Class is ready to start. I'm warmed up and ready and relieved to be here. Yesterday I drove the forty-five minutes to get to the gym but stayed out in the car, crying. I never made it in. Grief just overtook me. Sometimes I can't pull it together, so I let it fall apart. There's a certain serenity in letting things be as they are.

INQUIRY

Santa Cruz Mountains
August 2016

I used to keep an altar with some items that symbolized the peaceful mood of meditation laid out on a little wooden shelf. A candle, a Buddha, perhaps some flowers. Lighting the candle and settling into the cushion, I would begin the breathing technique or visualization I was working with at the time.

Nowadays I just have a cushion and an iPhone as a timer. No special items or pictures. I use a koan, a penetrating question, to help me find a sense of somatic energy. "Who am I?" I meditate with that question in the background, breath in the foreground. Thoughts and stories wash in and through me, like bits of flotsam washing in and out on shoreline waves. I notice I am reviewing a conversation and softly return attention to my own sense of present aliveness. *Who is this?* I query. A pang of guilt strikes, and I realize I just thought about my friend's birthday; I forgot to send a card. I return attention to my sense of "I." The waves of thought slow, lose velocity, get softer. My attention drops into a quieter place that feels solid.

"Who am I?" is a Zen question in the tradition of koans. It is also a contemplative question in the yoga tradition of inquiry. There are so many responses to this inquiry! We all have a natural sense of self, of identity, that marks us as separate from other creatures and things. Demarking a self is inherent in the most basic form of life. Separation from everything else by some kind of boundary is a precondition for life to persist. It occurred at the moment life began, by isolating the first protocell's replication machinery with a protective, permeable membrane. It recurs every time a cell membrane forms around a new daughter cell. The membrane actively defends the cell from predators and toxins. Each of the trillions of cells in our body is a fully separated life package.

At the same time, no cell or self is completely separate. Because the cell membrane is permeable, selected molecules pass in and out constantly. A cell is both separate from and intimate with everything around it.

Like a cell, I experience separation. I have a strong sense of being Rikki, a personality with opinions and preferences, judgments and sensitivities. Who is this Rikki? It seems like I am a coherent person, but upon deeper examination "I" appears more like a collection of voices than a solid person. It seems there is a mishmash of different selves; they arise, take care of some business, and fade away again. Are any of them me? Is my basic operating self just cobbled together from fragments? Am I just these various voices?

At first I thought this was the big deal—you realize your seemingly potent, impactful self is just a collection of thoughts. Satori! Nobody there! But that's not the interesting part. Somebody *is* there. Beneath all that noise, something *is* there. In meditation you can get an intuitive feel for this underneath being. Who am I behind these different voices and emotions? What persists while the content changes? There's a palpable vibrancy, a sense of impersonal potency. It is quiet, harmonious. This is a deeper, inclusive sense of expansive self. An energy that feels very stable yet fluid, welcoming to whatever arises. This is worth exploring. This is Rikki, too.

Like our cells, we are not completely separate. We also share a deep intimacy with our environment, each other, and other creatures. And we share experiences. Like other creatures, we feel joy and sadness, pride and shame. We all draw courage from the same well; we all find strength from the same inner source. We are all vulnerable to the same vicissitudes of life. This sharing we experience as love, with little or no feeling of separation between us. Love is expansive and not defensive; it's inclusive. But it takes courage to go beyond defensiveness into that deeper, loving, expansive self.

To find peace or freedom during the coming months with Linda, I will have to slow down and be present with whatever occurs. I can react from my separate sense of self, or I can find that place within where I am in harmony with what is. I can always breathe, and sometimes I will get a moment of choice. No one can grab that choice and make it for me. Inside, I am going to either seize the breakout moment or not; be the victim of my own confusion and ignorance or arouse my passion and intelligence to choose love. I am going to emerge from the narrow pass with an open, awake heart, or I am not.

HLA

Santa Cruz Mountains
Fall 2016

It takes nearly two months to complete the arrangements for donor viability tests and get all the results. I arrange appointments with my ob-gyn, the breast care center, my internist, and my colon doctor. The next few weeks are a blur. I finish the ob-gyn exam and endure the mammogram. Then I meet with my internist for a general physical and heart check. I schedule a colonoscopy. I use the time to build my strength and my intention to adjust my cellular markers.

My mammogram comes up with a shadow. A white windowed envelope with a bright pink notice inside blares at me from the kitchen counter. I don't even let the information in. I can't afford to even think about breast cancer. I have magical thinking: There is conservation of cancer; you get only so much in one family. Linda has taken on the whole thing. I am safe. Nonetheless, I open the envelope. They want me to come in for another test. I am just breathing in the upper half of my chest because I am scared. But I have to do it. I call to schedule the three-dimensional mammogram. Previously, I avoided this because I'll have to pay out of pocket, but now it's necessary. I take three slow, deep breaths just to show I remember how.

—

For a stem cell transplant, you want a donor who has identical cellular markers, called human leukocyte antigens (HLAs) for as many of the ten markers as possible. These ten markers are what your immune system uses to determine whether cells it encounters are good homies bearing the right tattoos or bad invaders from another 'hood. If you have the right markers, you get to live. If you have the wrong markers, your immune system prepares an attack on you.

These HLA markers are proteins. Proteins are long chains of carbon atoms with a few bright spots where other atoms link in. Each carbon atom in these long-chain molecules is not really a particle; it actually exists as a kind of potential energy, which buzzes along in neutral until it is poked to deliver a quantum of energy as a wave or particle, whichever the poker recognizes. When poked, one of these atoms pops a quantum of energy out of its vacuum long enough for it to interact with other atoms. You could say that all a wave or particle is is the form that the potential energy takes when it appears in space-time.

For example, when an active enzyme gets close enough to a protein, the enzyme transfers energy, as either particle momentum or wave frequency, to the protein. That energy twists the protein's shape. Just before they interacted, the enzyme and protein were in their potential energy state. The interaction causes them both to take form; then the enzyme's electromagnetic field interacts with the protein's and delivers energy that changes the protein's shape. It snaps from one position to another. The angles between the atoms change. Then everyone goes back to being in potential energy states until the next time they need to present a form. Everything is flipping in and out all the time: potential to form, forms interact, then back to potential.

The mathematics of these quantum behaviors are complicated. There is no good theory in physics to *explain* the behavior of these energy quanta. There are only equations to *predict* it. We don't know *why*, but we are sure that quantum mechanics, as equations and a set of predictions, is highly *correct*. So, according to quantum mechanics that underlies transistors (radios, processors, phones, cars) and lasers (CDs, DVDs) and all of chemistry, my entire being is made of vibrating energy that zings and pops in and out of form at light speed. Bits of energy exchange energy, always formatted as momentum or frequency. Then everything returns to a state of potential quantum energy.

Linda's markers have never been measured. Neither have mine. Who knows what value they have? We don't. And if they have never been measured, no one knows. It's a secret within our bodies. As far as the best science we have can tell me, the amazing fact is that our HLAs might be in any of their possible configurations. When the molecular configuration settled down to be measured, it would be determined, but the die was not yet cast. The possibility was open that we could be a 10/10 match.

I find a website that lists seven things you can do to enhance to the production of healthy stem cells, and I do them all:

- Cut sugar
- Reduce calories
- Reduce triglycerides
- Lift heavy weights and work out aerobically four times a week
- Take vitamins D_3 and E, curcumin, resveratrol, glucosamine, and chondroitin
- Stay at a slightly elevated altitude (I live at 2,200 feet)
- Avoid prescription medications

I get two of my doctors' attestations of my fitness to be a donor. I go down to the breast center again, and this time, I disrobe for the 3-D version of X-rays. My breasts are squashed, scrimped, and folded between the flattening plates; the cameras hum. We do this three or four times and the exam is complete. We shuffle me into the changing room again. "I'll have the doctor look at these right away. Just wait in here," the examiner tells me.

I remove the stickies from my breasts and get dressed, rocking on the edge of the changing bench while I wait. I wonder if the entity who examines the image is human or AI. I've been reading that AIs do a better job of finding patterns in data and have been producing more accurate diagnoses of cancers than trained cancer doctors. The AI could hide in a back room, treat the nurses with utter indifference, review hundreds of scans without getting tired or making errors, and never even need a cup of coffee.

Finally, the nurse returns and tells me the 3-D mammogram has verified that I do not have any suspicious spots. My ob-gyn gives her blessing to the donation.

Possible HLA match, check! Viable donor, check, check, check! I'll need two more checks in the viable-donor category—City of Hope and Kaiser will run extensive tests on me before we're finished. No worries there. During the remaining weeks, the more pressing issue for me will be this: Is there any way I can influence the outcome?

FIGHT FOR MYSELF

THE FAB FIFTIES
Santa Cruz Mountains
Fall 2016

Home in Santa Cruz, I make a rare phone call to check in with Linda or Rick. I send an occasional written note, a small gift, a charm for her charm bracelet. Text queries: "How's the nausea today? Feel like chess?" and "Are the test results in? How'd you do?" I keep track of dates and numbers. I just want her to know somebody is right there.

It's actually challenging to find the "caring without invading" sweet spot. Boundaries were confused in our family of origin; we kids were somehow responsible for our parents' welfare. Mother, ever at rope's end, blamed us for the most recent thing that pulled the rope. "See what you've done!" she would cry when Daddy threw something or started drinking during the daytime. "You know he needs that Coke. You should never ever drink the last Coke!" She was always sort of collapsing, and that might end with the Last Straw: someone (often me) getting shut out of the house or locked in the basement. All the insanity these two poor people made—it was all because they were drinking! If they hadn't been drinking, they would have had to grapple with their minds, at least to some degree. But that is not how they played it. They played it like the Fabulous Fifties.

—

Summer 1959

Iron-wheeled chaise lounges with thick water-resistant cushions stood among scattered red-striped towels and rubber thongs on the grass leading up to the pool. The pool was at the top of a little rise, about five feet, in the backyard of our home in Northbrook, a white-flight enclave north of Chicago. Uncle Jimmy crashed into the flat surface of the water on his back while Uncle Sonny hooted at him from above. The scent of barbecue lighter fluid and cigarettes wafted through the air. Crinkly packets of Camels and a sexy box of Benson & Hedges filters lay with silver-blue beer cans on the side tables next to crumpled paper napkins and Daddy's cocktail glass. Our huge, half-Olympic-size pool was squished out of its rectangle into a square. Daddy was telling the story of how the previous owner's wife, when the pool was first dug, snuck out in the middle of the night to move the stakes marking the dig site. Although I couldn't have been more than eight, I noted that the owner was male and that the female, to get what she wanted, successfully crept around in the dark.

My father was entertaining my uncles with one-liners. Uncle Bernie stretched out in a chaise longue, up on one elbow, drafting a Pabst Blue Ribbon. He laughed. Daddy was handsome and had an engulfing smile. His short, jet-black hair, wet from the pool, was combed back like Kookie's on *77 Sunset Strip*. He was the smartest, funniest, quickest man in any room. Everyone wanted his attention and talked to him first.

My uncles loved a good joke and a fun time. They were less complex than my father; they had not been to war. Their laughter was simpler and lacked the edge in my father's voice. It was like they were having a good time, whereas my father always had to have fun, be great, win admiration.

Mommy was laughing, waving a cigarette between two fingers

in a hand grasping a cocktail glass. The ice clinked. She was an unfeigned icon for the wife of an advertising executive. She was petite and kept her figure even after three childbirths. Her round cherub's face was shadowed by a wide-brimmed straw hat the color of clotted cream; the bangs and stray strands of her short bouffant peeked out and gave her an Audrey Hepburn look.

Great, woolly white cumulus clouds were heaped in the sky, promising an evening shower, but the sun was bright in early afternoon. In the summer heat, a bit of rain would be welcome but not cooling.

Sonny, Bernie, Jimmy—these were Mom's little brothers, probably her favorite people on earth. She wanted them to eat, to share the bounty of this envied life in the suburbs: a swimming pool in the backyard, a built-in barbecue on the patio, a screened-in porch for fleeing the mosquitoes on sweltering, humid July nights.

I was screaming, "Mommy Mommy Mommy look at me look at me!" while I did belly flops off the diving board. Bethy must have been on the blanket or taking a nap in a crib. She was a baby, not two yet.

Uncle Sonny was still a minor, but my father let him smoke cigarettes. Sonny packed Camels, but Dad was a Parliaments smoker. To each man, his own poison. Daddy liked scotch or gin martinis, but my uncles were just drinking beer. We didn't realize that drinking might affect Daddy's judgment. When he was regular Daddy, he was charming and warm and we all wanted to be in his love sphere. Whenever he sang the old ditty "He's Got the Whole World in His Hands" in his happy, booming baritone, he made us feel safe and protected.

One time, he let Linda fly out the back of Mother's Oldsmobile convertible into the street behind us. One minute, we were sitting side by side with Leslie Pollack on the back of the rear seat of the white Olds with the top down, cruising on the boulevard, cool as any kids on vacation. Daddy hummed that red-leathered baby up to a red light and let it rumble. Then, when the light greened, he put the car in drive and moved out—and Linda tumbled, heels over head, onto the roadside.

We yelled, "Linda's out! Linda's out!" When he heard, he jammed the car to a stop. Looking over his shoulder, he reversed, threw it in park, jumped out, and ran to her. Confused, she was wandering through traffic to the curb. Daddy picked her up and carried her to the car. He made a joke of it; he made a joke of her. Maybe that was the first time he called her Lady Roundheels. There was something wrong with that phrase and we all knew not to tell Mom. But did I tell Mom anyway? I was unreliable. I lacked impulse control.

There was a green martini glass painted on the bottom of the pool, about six feet tall and a couple feet across. A toothpick the size of a broom handle punctured the softball-size green olive at the bottom of the glass. I have a definite memory of something red. Was there a red pimento in the olive?

Each spring we drained the yucky water and repainted the surface. The winter weather dumped tons of leaves and debris, but for some reason we did not cover the pool, maybe because it was an odd shape, or too large. The dreaded cleaning and painting ritual was laborious, and these uncles often showed up to help with the hard part. One year, after we vacationed in California, we returned home to Northbrook, where Mom's brothers were taking care of the house. They were telling Dick they'd come over next weekend and help get the pool cleaned up if he wanted, when we walked over to look at the mess and found—surprise!—they had done it all while we were gone, and it was already filling with clear water.

The martini glass was missing that year. In a normal year, a freshly painted martini glass was the handiwork of family friend Annie Snyder, to whose home we escaped with Mom on occasion when Daddy was violent. Annie loved to drink as much as anyone and had convinced my parents that this symbol of our lifestyle at the bottom of our pool was no shame but a call to action! Drink on, merry pranksters. The pool was just one of the things that made managing the Northbrook property a Problem that sparked Daddy to overdrink. Otherwise, Daddy drank just for fun. Life is but a dream.

But life was not dreamy for my father, whose drinking was already, when he was still younger than thirty-five, a consuming, desperate, endless cycle. Daddy would get louder and turn mean if he stayed on course that afternoon. Mom had to get things going on the barbecue. Uncle Bernie helped her. Although he, too, would become an alcoholic, he was one who would get sober in AA. They balanced the loosening effect of booze with the stabilizing effect of steaks, potato salad, Coca-Cola, boiled artichokes with mayo-lem-on-mustard dip, and deviled eggs. I made the artichoke dip. Uncle Bernie put the steaks on. Linda helped with the deviled eggs.

Next to the pool was a half-acre apple and pear orchard, with a long row of mature grapes purpling on the vines that crawled the cyclone fencing around the pool. Linda had decamped to the shade under an apple tree with a book. I wanted attention. My friend Alan and I had laboriously hammered a small platform, a fanciful tree house, in one of the apple trees. I leaped out of it onto the ground below. "I am Superman! Look at me! Look at me!" I clambered back up. Linda regarded me with disapproval and relocated to a quieter spot, closer to the adults. I was suddenly isolated and cut off. I climbed down and went out to the driveway to kick rocks.

By the time the fellows drove off in Bernie's VW bug, Daddy was drunk—uncontrollable, stumbling around the house, shouting and muttering. God willing, he would pass out early. He gibbered when he was drunk. He attacked Mommy for nothing—for being a bitch, for nagging him. I wonder if he got her confused with his mother, because once he did smash everything in the house that belonged to his mother, along with the vigorous fighting bulls my mother collected.

Mom picked these bulls up on vacations after becoming enamored of bullfighting in Mexico—or, rather, of the vitality and energy of the sleekly muscled Spanish fighting bull and the sexy bravado of the matador. She acquired ceramic bulls in every posture of charging ferocity, and they stippled our shelves. Daddy smashed them all. Only one of Mommy's bulls survived; it's not ceramic. It's cast-iron, heavy. I'm holding it in my hand at this moment. It's small, taut, stylized, powerful—a real Picasso of a charging bull.

Intermingled in our living room were beautiful antique gas lamps, modified for electric bulbs, belonging to Daddy's now-dead mother, Nonni, left over from when she and Granddaddy lived in this house. Daddy smashed them, too. By the time I realized my father might have his own childhood nightmares, he was dead and gone; I could not ask about them. And after the night of the Big Smash, these exhibits of his entanglement were no longer in our care.

But this was not that night. I ran around outside among the trees and shadows until Mother remembered she had children and told me to come in. She must have put Elizabeth to bed already, because she did not ask Linda to do it. Linda went to her room to find her own comforts—music or poetry, I suspect. I played with my cap guns: a six-shooter and a Winchester rifle. Linda had the small upstairs room at the rear corner of the house until Bethy's birth, a year ago November. Now she had the downstairs room with the bay window. No, that was later. In 1959 we shared the big upstairs front room. Yes, we had the pair of single beds, and the antique desk that belonged to Nonni, under which our secret clubhouse for stuffed animals lay hidden in our imagination.

This was not the night that I baited the bear and he came after me to kill me and I locked myself in the upstairs bathroom, which had a way out onto the roof of the breezeway, which was not high at all. I could easily jump down. Later in life, when I saw *The Shining*, I would remember that night with far more terror than I felt at the time. Elizabeth and I agreed that Jack Nicholson did such a good rendition of raging drunk Daddy that he nauseated us both.

This was not the night that Linda called the cops because Daddy was going to kill someone, but when they arrived, Bethy and I were sitting on the stairs in our jammies and Linda was standing in the doorway to the den. Mom said everything was fine, no problems here; Daddy had passed out in the den. This was not any of those nights.

We put ourselves to bed, brushing our teeth and tumbling ourselves into our jammies. If we were lucky, Daddy would be asleep when Mom came in to say good night. If not, there would be arguments. He would start to call her names, whore and cunt and whatnot; she could go either way, attacking him and fighting back or collapsing in tears.

Linda liked to play the portable RCA record player Granddaddy gave her for her birthday. She would put on the 33-rpm Broadway album *The Music Man* while she drifted off, but the last song on the first side, a slow melody that was probably a love song, gave me the creeps. I hurried to get to sleep before it started.

QUEST
Santa Cruz Mountains
Fall 2016

"Alexa," I tell the round disc on the windowsill, "play Bach's unaccompanied Cello Suites by Yo-Yo Ma." She does.

Taa, la de da da da da dum, taa la de da da da da dum—the repeated opening phrase of Suite No. 1 is immediately soothing. The cello's vibration in my chest quiets my racing thoughts. I take two slow, full breaths in and out.

I woke from restless sleep feeling lost. I am ashamed to be so healthy. Our fragile vulnerability frightens me. To stay steady I must navigate a private path through an inner maze. For perhaps the first time, my sister is the one in need. I have to stand up inside so I can show up. I have to connect with the thing in me that I can count on.

I have these tools: Yoga. American Zen. 12 Steps. Despite their wildly different language, each of these transformational frameworks offers me some perspective and tools for dealing with my inner life. Yoga teaches me how to work with energy in the body and breath. Zen helps me get real and honest about what is actually present and alive, versus feel-good concepts. The 12 Steps give me the basic framework for sanity: Let go of control and let a higher, deeper power manage the future. Take responsibility for the consequences of my behavior and choices now.

To calm my mind, I do alternate-nostril breathing. This is a yoga breath technique that helps create a steady, stable state of mind, at least for the moment, and that is where I am. I pinch my nose shut gently, then open the right side to inhale for a count of four. Then I close up, count to eight, and open the left side to exhale for eight. I repeat on the other side, then do the whole thing again three more times.

This exercise does a couple of things: First, because you are withholding breath, the mind pays attention quickly. It is very attentive to its survival. In this technique, you count, creating a rhythm that makes it easy to concentrate. You narrow your spotlight of attention to the breath, rather than opening to the ebb and flow of whatever arises. It's like changing the focus in a camera lens. Second, the long exhale gets rid of carbon dioxide so the percentage of oxygen in the blood can rise. Now, at least for a few seconds, my mind is calming down. My trains of thought have been derailed. I can start fresh.

I imagine a simple, quiet, restful energy in the center of my body. Breathing slowly, I focus light attention on the sense of "I am" right in my solar plexus. Just the feeling of being. This feeling of being can be difficult to discern. It took me years of meditation before I noticed it. I guess I was looking for something unusual. But the energy of life and clarity of intuition are ordinary. There is nothing special about them. I attend to the feeling of aliveness in the middle of me. I remember that this links me to the energy that I can count on, and that I connect with it in meditation. I can't connect right now, but I remember. I remember I can trust that thing I trust to feed me whatever I need in the way of courage, patience, compassion, and Mother's kindness.

As a kid, I wanted to discover something that would save my parents from their confusion and unhappiness. Where would I find that?

Linda was the smart one. Bethy was barely a toddler. I was not very virtuous. I cheated at games and took the last cookies and blamed Bethy. I'd lie if I needed to. I'd steal. I'd try to find the easier, softer way. Who was I to save my parents?

The world in the 1960s seemed to be a place of confusion and unhappiness. My generation of white boomers flourished in the soil of complaint about the injustice, stupidity, and flatness of life in Good America after the war. Pete Seeger and Bob Dylan were our folk heroes; the beat poets and French existentialists defined the emotional landscape. Kennedy symbolized the liberal dream of globalizing democracy. The civil rights conflict got uglier and more polarized daily. The Vietnam War, a mortal sin, permanently damaged the moral position of the "free" world and eroded our decency. Science made clear that it had abandoned its job of finding truth: Its job had become engineering, not knowledge. Quantum mechanics had bumped space, time, and causality into a hopeless pile of quaint ideas and left nothing—literally a vacuum—in its place. Our world offered no justice, no order, no boss, no structure, no purpose beyond consumption and pleasure. My hippie clan sought redemption for ourselves and blamed our parents' generation. We imagined the grown-ups knew what they were doing. But I knew my parents were lost.

A sense of desperation floods me. Can we do anything at all to help other people? But it was not my job to save my parents from their destiny. In reality I'll be lucky to work out my own salvation.

MY LIFE IS MY ART
Santa Cruz Mountains
Fall 2016

But what does it even mean to work out your own salvation? The phrase echoes with the sound of little Catholic footsteps trudging down the hall to the office of Mother Superior. I was terrified of that woman, but I wonder: Did she find our shenanigans more amusing than she let on? How horrid could we really be, a bunch of eight-year-olds in navy jumpers with short-sleeved white shirts bearing soft, buttoned Peter Pan collars? But apparently we were horrid enough to require discipline, and that's what I faced at St. Norbert's. A rap on the knuckles with a ruler? Standing in the corner? Just being glared at by that bear of a woman was enough. When I was upset, I goofed around. I was never going to get myself under control at school while things were crazy at home.

We uniformed souls were taught to seek our salvation through prayer and the sacraments of the Church. We attended Mass at least once during the week. If I was lucky, we would sing. My grammy on Mom's side used to take me to church with her on Sunday mornings if Mom let me sleep over. She beamed her heart to god's ears. I loved to sing to god with her. You could really open your throat and let your being be out there. Otherwise, you had to button it all up.

None of us girls in our sturdy cordovan loafers with their shining copper pennies thought of ourselves as souls seeking god's forgiveness. We felt like wild things, vibrant troublemakers, tree climbers and merry-go-rounders. Much later I learned of the Buddha's suggestion of finding out for yourself. Try various methods to discern how your own mind works, to excavate your own freedom, and to unleash your compassion. That is the path for wild things. At sixty-five, I am still a tree climber and merry-go-rounder. I want to know myself honestly and tap my authentic energy before I die.

Linda once told me my life is my art. My paintbrush and sketch pencil are my intentions; my muse is trust. I set an intention, like a broad sweep of the brush, to orient myself to the possibilities in that direction.

Setting an intention helps me see and make choices that are aligned with it. You don't just appear magically out of nothing; you fabricate yourself out of your possibilities, either by reacting or by aligning with intentions. You hit times in life when you need courage, and you pull it out of nowhere if you have the intention to get through it. Somehow you get to AA, quit drinking, and work the 12 Steps. Sometimes unconscious patterns drive you and you find a good therapist to help you untangle the mess. Or you don't. The question is: Am I able to choose, or do the patterns take over?

Having clear intentions helps me see choices that encourage them to become reality. Setting an intention is like sliding a curling stone; it sets a trajectory and creates a set of possibilities. I can influence my curling-stone trajectory significantly with intelligent and vigorous sweeping—my in-the-moment choices. If I am present, instead of triggered, I get a moment of choice. When I am completely clouded by fear or anger or whatever, I have no space to make any choices. I just wave my broom over my head, forgetting to sweep.

Being on a trajectory enables me to see potential choices consistent with the aspiration. Mistakes and setbacks will happen, but the intention is bigger than any errant sweeps. I don't have to let a reactive pattern take control. And it's great to watch my choices bring my intention into the world.

I have a big short-term intention to be a perfect stem cell donor for Linda. The first challenge is the miracle of being a match. The extraction process itself will not ask too much of me. It will be like a marathon blood donation. I'll take a drug that stimulates stem cell production, and they will filter the stem cells out of my blood in a process similar to dialysis. They estimate it will take two six-hour sessions. The challenge for me is somehow to be an HLA match and then to produce the fattest, healthiest, most well-intentioned stem cells imaginable.

And I have a big long-term intention—call it an aspiration—to see through my delusions for the sake of all beings. Even my dog.

I whistle and call her name. "Hey, Zoey. Want to go for a walk?" Zoey likes to spend most of her sleep time on the bed, tangled in her blue plaid blanket. Part American Staffie and part coyote, with some little lap dog mixed in, she is willing to open an eye to watch me, but she won't invest more energy than that quite yet. Her eye follows me across the room, alert to whether I step toward the closet where I keep my hiking sneakers. If we are going out, I will get those and sit on the stairs to put them on. Sure enough, I open the closet door. She leaps off the bed, body eager, ears up, focused intently. I grab the black-and-purple sneakers, and she barks and leaps in a little circle. When I sit down on the top step of the staircase and start to put them on, she's licking my face and hopping about. "Woof!" We trundle down the full flight of stairs, bumping into each other, landing in the kitchen.

She heads to the garage door, then looks back at me when she reaches the step. Are we going? "Yes," I say, nodding, and she prances to the door. Then she comes back to the pantry and looks at me, looks at the pantry. Looks at me, wags her tail. If we're going on a trail walk, I will get some treats, and she knows this. "Okay, I'll get some treats," I say, and at the word *treats*, her tail wags double-time. I get the stash and move toward the garage door, then retrace my steps to fetch a leash from the hall closet. She runs after me and watches from the kitchen. She is able to read my body language, and she stays attentive so she knows what's coming next.

We do go out the door, and she runs ahead. At the end of the driveway, she looks back. Are we going? If I say, "No, no, no. No walks for dogs today," she will come back. If I say, "Yes! Yes, we're really going," she will trot into the private road.

Zoey definitely has the ability to hold an intention. It seems like her intentions are variations of presets, like instincts, such as "stay attuned to my human." She also intends to chase squirrels, to convince me to brush her coat, and to get the marrow out of her chew bone. But, as far as I can tell, she can't intend to awaken from ignorance for the sake of all beings. To set a completely new intention and ask that your whole organism reorganize around that intention seems to be a special opportunity afforded to a human brain.

I want the benefits of my intention to enliven my holistic inner self to spread out in the world through the six degrees of separation. Everyone who comes into contact with my vibrations will benefit from a clearer, happier Rikki. I'm not willing to be driven by unconscious patterns anymore. I am putting up a fight. I want my curling stone humming on the ice path of accessing my authentic, whole self, not just for me but for the sake of all beings.

I easily see how my unconscious and sometimes destructive patterns get triggered by other people's unconscious triggered reactions, to the point that we get tangled up in each other's patterns and are unable to escape. I'm motivated to help us all get out of this mess. That bit of freedom lets everyone in my drivetrain be free of the extra torque. And, as my friend Illana says, even a little freedom is still freedom.

I sense intuitively that my life is part of a greater whole, one inner world in which we all participate. Science tells me a similar thing about the physical world: From my understanding of the Copenhagen interpretation of quantum physics, I gather that there is—in quantum reality—one interconnected, quantum state of the whole universe each moment of its appearance. In Buddhism, they call this "dependent arising," because everything is connected to, and dependent on, everything else.

On a smaller scale, there is certainly one interconnected life here on earth that is continually sharing energy back and forth. That energy is never created or destroyed; it just changes form. The vibes over here in my neck of the woods are not separate from the vibes in yours, though we may sometimes seem light-years apart. We are like waves in the sea. We influence and are influenced. We are like a Twitter community. I'd like to see intention and compassion trending.

To stick with an intention takes trust. You have to trust that there is more to life than can be seen with ordinary, foggy vision, and that life is working for you in the background—that you can tune in to that beneficial energy with your intuition. I am trusting that we are going to be carried through this somehow. I am not one to believe; I don't take anything on faith. Then again, I can be a sucker for the Answer or the Truth, since I am so hungry for it. But when I look carefully and deeply at what has pulled me through in bad times, I find my heart trusts. Secretly I trust my own life to make sense and find its way to something worthwhile.

During the hard times when I was so very down and out and alone, I always felt like there was a Way Through. No matter how dark things were, I knew that couldn't be the end of the story. Something will always rise out of the depths, somehow. If you must, you will meet all the gargoyles, but you will find what is on the other side of despair. Trust will pull you through.

Sometimes, to find the energy inside you that you can trust, you have to give up a lot of stuff that you think defines you—stuff you think is important: your pride, your daydream, something; your arrogance, your credentials, your reasons for being better than others. But there is definitely something inside that you can trust to make the right choice for you. Every time, it can choose your well-being over "looking good" or showing off your credentials. After years of practicing the 12 Steps and meditating, I connected with this willingness. There I was, with the intention to choose my own well-being. What a joy to find something I could trust in myself! There is great freedom in that.

The *content* of my mind is often confused and chaotic. If you listen in, you'll hear criticism, defensiveness, and striving to look good. But you can also discern the uplifting impulse to be free, the impulse to know, the impulse to love. Those impulses come from somewhere and are connected to something. Underneath the noise, I trust that somehow, in the depths, my own mind contains the source it seeks. I intend to connect with that. Trusting in the dark, I stumble through my own maze, marking the walls with my intuition penknife. These are the ways I work out my salvation.

In the deepest quiet of your private imaginings, don't you sense there is something in your life that is worth discovering? A treasure of incomparable value? That sense of our inner worth is what makes people yearn for justice, for things to turn out well for the underdog; for heavens and bright futures and fix-all technologies. We know there is something powerful in us. It seems to me that the treasure is right here in me as a mysterious aliveness and vitality. It's just very hard to discern.

Linda and I make arrangements with the people at City of Hope. They will send me a donor test kit. She already has several searches going on stem cell donor databases like Be The Match. It's fall already. Soon she will start infusions of the chemotherapy drugs known as R-CHOP (rituximab, cyclophosphamide, Hydroxydaunomycin, Oncovin, prednisone).

MAGIC MARKERS

MIND MOVES

Mountain View
Fall 2016

I arrive early at the gym, before the night class. Long black leather bags hang in a row along a mirror like sentries waiting for action. In the empty gym, they call out to be punched and kicked; we are going to work ourselves up to great things on these bags. The mat still smells more like Pine-Sol than like funk; the cleaners have just left. In a couple of hours, the mats and air will be rank with all our feet and sweat and battered equipment scattered around, but the dozens of us who cram onto the mat and into the ring don't care. Sweat is honorable here.

Jake is looking cool in white, gold, and red Thai shorts. My body is sore from workouts, and I'm crabby. I'm hoping we'll skip jumping rope today and go right to shadowboxing.

"Grab a rope; we'll get it going," booms Jake, in his big, friendly way.

My heart tries to sink a little, but I can't afford to lose the lift, so I perk up and jog over to grab a rope. We use a thick, weighted nylon rope, which helps the rope stretch out even though I'm not whipping it with the speed of the young athletes around me. I roll my shoulders back a few times, forward twice. I don't jump until I hear the buzzer. The first minute, two minutes, are easy. I go slowly and set a good rhythm. You see boxers in a gym whipping that cord around with crossed arms and hopping on different feet—that's not me. I whip at maybe two-thirds their pace, sometimes one-half, so I can stay in sync with the music beat.

By the third round, I expect to have a heart attack and am pleased with myself. What a great place to die. Everyone will talk about how I went out swinging—literally swinging that rope around. Jump. Jump. I count to calm my mind. Sets of four. One, two, three, four. One, two, three, four. It's like all you ever have to do is this one number; the others take care of themselves. I stare at the crack where the glass of the mirror meets the mat.

We work with focus mitts after I warm up on the bag. Jake holds the mitts up in front of his chest and calls out the strikes he wants me to make. "One!" is the jab. "One! Two!" is jab-cross. "Three" is the left hook. There's also a "six," which means jab-cross-hook-cross-upper-cut-cross. If you hit effectively, you will have your feet planted, your weight shifting, and your strike snappy. I throw a series of strikes. "Loosen your hands. Snap the punches out." As with everything in life, it's important to relax your muscles so the punch can swing with full force, tightening up just at the end to drive all the power into one snap. Unnecessary tension just wastes energy and tires you out.

Now I regret I haven't spent more time standing on one leg, strengthening my balance. "Put up a hard block! Harden your core." To block an incoming kick, you have to be able to stand on one leg. I'm standing on my rear leg and lift my left in front of me, bent at the knee, foot flexed, to block the incoming right kick. "Make your stance hard. When he kicks your leg, it hurts. You stay balanced, and he's hurt. He'll think before he does it again." Jake simulates a kick in slo-mo; I harden my core and raise my left to block. He taps my shin with his toe, and my leg wobbles. What an embarrassment!

Jake holds the mitts over my head for the last thirty seconds of the set. I punch one-two continuously. My mind is screaming whining sounds. I push past that, no extra energy, just punch-punch-punch *it is okay to die here* punch-punch-punch. "Good job!" he says at the buzzer. I walk it off. I breathe through my nose. I am always ready.

"Got another round in you?"

Of course. What else can you say to Jake? And anyway, I am here to meet my mind. I watch it wish Jake had not said that. I bolster myself with my voice. "Of course I do!"

Just shouting raises some energy I can use. You wouldn't believe how much you can go through in three minutes, or in eight sets of three minutes each. Frustration flashes when you miss a shot, stumble, fail to block. Anger flashes when he teases. *Of course you're stronger, dickwad,* I think.

I hit a series of jab-cross-hooks and hear, "Nice job, Rikki." And I believe him and feel gigantic. A real fighter. I want to jab-cross-hook all day, but we have moved to "Body hooks!" and I go: Pivot left, hook. Pivot right, hook. Pivot, hook. Thirty seconds, bam-bam-bam. You get into a rhythm slamming the whole body as a unit, from feet through hips and core to shoulders, moving to "slam the door" as the right or left hook slams into the belly pad he wears around his middle. "Ten more seconds!" Jake calls out to encourage me, but it lasts for twenty at least. "Good job!" We're done.

Instantly my mind relaxes, I flush with satisfaction and pride, and there is, for now, nothing else anywhere I should be doing. I'm just doing this, and I am awesome! Is this enlightenment?

When you stay with yourself longer than you thought you could, when you find yourself still there for you when you thought you had given up, you find yourself rising to meet you. You discover that there might be courage or forgiveness or self-compassion right when you need them. You think you are exhausted, but your own life rises up like a yoga breath, filling all the spaces. Some years ago, in the worst of my depression during joblessness, when I felt most alone in the world, my own heart rose up to meet me. I heard my own voice calling out from the depths, "I have always been here for you." Since then I've been certain, without being able to understand, that there is something within waiting to catch me when I am ready to give in and relax. That something is an intangible mystery; a vitality that underlies the appearance of everything; a vibrant, unending yearning to be, to know, and to embrace. It's my fathomless life. I don't know what it is, but awareness of it is like having a best friend or discovering half a million dollars in your bank account. It feels stable and sane and centered.

I take a few mouthfuls of water and run my head under the cold-water faucet. It's hard for my postmenopausal form to throw off all the heat. Fortunately, my body has learned to sweat more now, to cool me down more. I get a one-minute rest period before we start the Muay Thai drills. That will add kicks, elbows, knees, and blocks to the combinations.

Jake straps the Thai pads to his forearms. He'll hold these off to his side for me to kick. "On the ball of your foot!" Jake nods at my planted foot. "From the hips. Bring the shoulders. Up on the foot."

One. Two. Three. I kind of hate him right now. Step out to the right; swing the left leg up and straight across, leading with the hip and shoulder, up onto the ball of the right foot as it pivots. Five, six, seven. Keep the right glove up by my temple. And, finally, "You got this. Nine. Ten. Take a break. Good job!"

We do a set of three three-minute rounds with kicks, teeps, knees, elbows, blocks. I am just throwing my body parts at the pads by the time we are done, just laughing and empty. "Awesome, Rikki! You are so strong!"

Yes! is all I can think. It's all I have left.

On the way home, I road-rage at people just like me trying to get home. Is there no rest for this mind?

MIND OVER HLA?
Santa Cruz Mountains
Fall 2016

Since the HLA molecules are part of my body, can my thoughts influence them? Do my thoughts influence molecules in my body? Surely they do. I think; therefore, I move. I am thinking as I type, and lots of molecules are involved in making that happen. Thoughts occur as signals in the brain material, and, just around the time the thought *lift my arm* occurs, my arm lifts. Apparently, a thought caused a signal. Is it only brain molecules that thoughts can influence?

No one has any idea how thoughts in a mind empower an arm to move. We can trace the neurons and see it happen, but where is the thought experienced? Where is the person, or the choice? Nobody has a clue where you are or where the choice is. You just intend for something like *lift leg* to happen, and it happens. No one knows where the intention is or how it arises.

The way we absently think about it is the way it came to us from European thinking centuries ago, which saw the mind as part of a disembodied soul. At some point in physical development, this soul was supposed to enter the body and manage it from there on, particularly mastering the body's sinfulness. But those ideas are out-dated. Nowadays, the best science suggests that the mind is magically produced by the complexity of patterns of synchronized circuitry in the frontal-parietal area of the brain, with no central agent or person in there. There is no little person, like a soul, who makes choices and directs attention. Most decisions happen unconsciously; we know about them after they are a done deal. This is why I am never surprised when I find myself eating ice cream the same evening I thought I swore off it. Yet we certainly experience being that soul or central agent. It's very unsatisfying to think about this, because you go in circles. I am right here, asking questions about how there is someone here asking questions when there is no place where she might be.

But in real life, however it works, I can raise my arm; I can move my body. I can hold my breath; I can slow my heartbeat. I can run and sing. So some molecules in my body are intimately related to some of my thoughts. Some molecules in my body follow the direction of certain thoughts; let's call these intentions. Intentions have a kind of directed energy that moves arms and directs attention.

In real life, intentions make a real difference and cause real things to happen. I intend lots of things, short- and long-term. I intend to update the software on my iPad, and I intended to become pregnant. Having a clear intention brings to the fore opportunities and choices that can shape the available options in my life. If some unconscious pattern does not block me, I can make choices that align with my intentions.

What I don't know is, can my intentions influence tiny molecules in my own body if they are not connected to my brain? Is my brain connected to all the parts in my body, even the cells? I can feel the slight pain of a miniscule paper cut; it seems like my brain is pretty connected to tiny rips in my fingertip. How do intentions in my brain influence my tissues, cells, and molecules?

Many people believe prayer influences outcomes, but how would that happen? How are my thoughts, presumably encoded in brain signals, going to influence anything even inches away from my cerebral cortex? Can we influence the vibration of energies that are not physically in contact with us? How would the influence be transmitted? Does proximity matter in the world of energies and quanta? Can influence be transmitted over distance without contact?

Well, yes, actually, influence *can* be transmitted over distance without contact. Science can replicate that strange phenomenon in very special situations. It turns out that proximity is not always necessary in the quantum world. In certain experiments, information can be transmitted instantly over distance without contact, without time for the information to travel from here to there. Nobody has a testable theory of reality to explain this strange fact, that causality among quanta is sometimes nonlocal. Physicists can witness a particular quantum event here and see that it "causes" a *simultaneous* event there. The cause was *here*, and, without traveling through space over time to deliver the cause, the effect happened *there*.

Of course, I can't draw any conclusions from these kinds of experiments. We don't know what they mean; we just know that they upend our brick-and-mortar universe of solid objects. And they have left many open questions and some contradictions in physics.

We are left with the situation that *we don't understand* how causality really works underneath the covers, in the quantum world, where we actually exist as popping energy. We have models for causality at the level of objects, but not at the level of quanta. Nor have we any models at the level of thought. We don't know how thoughts influence matter. If we don't really understand, there's no point believing in outdated physical ideas. We used to think only local contact had causal influence; now we don't know. Let's be honest. Western culture tells me it's silly to think my thoughts can impact my body, but I think, *Not so fast. Some thoughts do. I'm keeping an open mind.*

I'm in a situation where I don't know. The best science does not clarify the answer; in fact, science has exposed areas of dumbfounded ignorance. Zen is completely agnostic on these kinds of questions. Zen is interested only in the healthiness of your awareness. Yoga suggests the universe is full of energies and that the material world is somewhat fluid, which is intriguing but not specific. I want to have faith that my intention will have influence, but it's a gamble. Here's what I think I know: Thoughts are embodied as brain states. Brain states do influence physical activity in the body by sending signals along pathways. My intention starts a stream of events that result in my arm moving. Could my intention start a stream of events that result in my having a 10/10 HLA match with my sister? I don't know.

INSANE EXPERIMENT, NO CONTROL

Santa Cruz Mountains
Fall 2016

An insane experiment, but unavoidable: I have trouble imagining being alive in a world without my older sister. We are survivors of a traumatic childhood. We are like soldiers who kept each other sane and alive through deadly combat together. When we were kids, we named our parents Laugh a Minute (Mom) and Crazy Horse (Dad) to try to get some perspective on the distressed state of their lives. We spoke in a secret language and tried to keep our footing as our parents' world tilted in the wind.

Once, after visiting an art museum in London, Linda got a print of a portion of a John Singer Sargent painting and had it framed for me. It shows two buoyant, hand-holding girls in an English garden, poised to chase a tantalizing butterfly into unknown shrubbery. The younger girl is heedlessly racing off to new discoveries; the older pulls back a bit, recommending caution.

I talk to that Linda in my head all the time. She is, I fantasize with an adolescent attitude, the person who most deeply understands and cares about me, like a substitute parent. Doesn't she want to know what book I am reading, what heartache stained my weekends?

After our dramatic fight last April, though, I had to take on board the idea that she maybe had a different experience. Maybe she didn't relish having a little sister. Maybe I burdened her with expectations that she play a role that wasn't hers to play. I was beginning to understand how my parents' pains impacted the forming of a self within me. Certainly, Linda faced the same young challenges. Did she, too, feel isolation, abandonment, shame? Anyway, maybe screaming for attention makes me come off like a jerk.

But here we are in a real life-and-death situation. What does being or not being a jerk have to do with it? I know I have to come up with a 10/10 match and that my deepest intentions might have something to do with the outcome. I choose to trust.

You know how it is to watch a basketball player pull a magnificent performance out of nothing in the last minutes of some critical quarter? You know the feeling of being there when a freestyle blues guitarist runs spontaneous riffs that carry everyone to a new place? There's a zone thing. There's a way in which every muscle fiber and every thought is attuned and every emotion is focused—lightly, but absorbed—and then the fingers go, the body is aligned, everything just happens like it was easy. I need to be in the zone, focused on being a perfect match. I can't help it; in my deepest heart, I keep repeating, *Please be a match, please be a match. I know you can do it; it's all energy; please just do that for us.*

I have no way of knowing whether my galvanized intention can influence the state of my molecules to match an unknown quantity. But maybe. Because I suspect my being is not isolated and solitary any more than my body is isolated and solitary. Because I suspect my being is coequal to all being, comprising all beings. Because I suspect the wisdom in me—including the impenetrable secrets of life and evolution embedded in my own cells—may be able to handle this sort of thing. How can you know these things for sure? I have to trust it.

I know I have to keep meditating. Staying on course requires an intuitive, heartfelt practice as the foundation, like nutrition and sleep for the body. I am looking to stay balanced, in the flow, in the zone. I could easily get out of balance, believing fantasies of healing power, or fantasies of failure, or variations on these that have little to do with reality but that would throw the energies, unconscious and conscious, into disarray. As Chögyam Trungpa Rinpoche used to say, when you relate to reality, it is very simple, but if you start getting heroic or trying to prove something, it's dangerous. Your unconscious patterns throw you off, and it's hard to stay honest. I use meditation as a prophylactic every day.

It seems that when I am in the zone or flow, my energy engages the world smoothly and things just work out easily. I pick up the magazine with the article that has just the tip I need, or I get the check I've forgotten about that was lost in the mail. The flow state deactivates self-criticism from the prefrontal lobe and minimizes fear from the amygdala, allowing a kind of natural intelligence to guide me. It allows me to be intimate with the world, exchanging information freely, without as much background patter. And, like the intelligence in cells, it is mysterious to my human mind.

I don't know how it works, but it is real. You *feel* yourself moving rhythmically through the world, bumping into something you were looking for. Magically, the ideas you need for the paper you are writing are there for you. At the gym, your rhythm is great and your body feels smoothly coordinated. You are in sync; your timing is on; life is good. That lasts for a few days sometimes. But does that work over weeks or decades? Could just being in the flow guide a longer arc? Can you stay in the flow long enough to be where you need to be and go where you need to go, before you know what you need to do?

I suspect yes, but I can't see how inner mystery shapes my life. You have to listen in silence, and trust.

I want my whole being—my neuromuscular system and all the thoughts and emotions—aligned with the same intention. I don't want any unconscious patterns—which by definition I cannot yet know about—to undermine this effort. I will make the most focused possible intention and beam it continuously from my heart until I get the report. I am already fighting for myself; now I can fight for both of us.

And I don't resent the effort. It does a body a ton of good to stop listening to all its issues and complaints, judges and critics, worriers and blamers. For these months, I focus on a single intention, balanced through meditative practice. I'm in the zone.

The concentration enables me to rest in silence. Something different begins to happen in my inner world. Rather than always being jumbled by the negative and fractured patterns stored in my system, I find that silence calms me. That lets me sense myself differently. Something begins to shift the broken child's unconscious patterns to the side. Rather than feeling isolated, as I often do in my thoughts, in silence I connect to a web of friendly energy. There is just something familiar there that welcomes me. It feels like visiting friends at an oasis filled with food and water. In this comforting warmth, a wholeness and freedom grow quietly in me. I feel calm and complete within myself. I feel ready to be present without needing to be reassured or comforted, or even to be reassuring or comforting. I'm just present with it, whatever it is.

Mustering a shift like this takes passion, focus, and commitment that I have not marshaled for myself. I can rally it only for my sister Linda. It's always been easier for me to do something for someone else than to do it for myself. Yet the gifts that come are all for me.

INTUITION
Santa Cruz Mountains
Fall 2016

"Why are you in my kitchen when I'm cooking?" I whine at Jill. "Out out out!" I splatter the air with tiny, shining droplets of shallot-lemon-butter sauce from my dripping wooden spoon.

"Hey! It's not your kitchen." Jill, who understandably does not want sauce on her blouse, reaches out to stop my hand. She has just come in from work and is putting something in the garbage compactor, which is right in the middle of everything. I'm feeling crowded. Sometimes she starts cleaning while I'm still cooking. Utensils in use have disappeared without warning. Today she is innocent, but I am irritable. "What is wrong with you?" she queries.

Indeed, what *is* wrong with me? "Nothing. What's wrong with *you*?" I say, but I think, *You just walk in here like it's a family kitchen!* though I realize that makes no sense. Then it strikes me that I'm in a State. I am Off. Which is Understandable. Instead of fighting with Jill, I could acknowledge what is going on with me. I'm walking around in a daze. I'm not ready for Linda to die. *Die!* I am only sixty-five; I don't even have her grand-niece or grand-nephew yet. I need to steady my mind. Things are happening on multiple levels; I am scared for Linda, my sister and friend. I am scared for me, losing my lifelong friend. I am disturbed by this confrontation with death. Death ends things so completely. It really reshuffles your deck.

Outside our kitchen window runs the expanse of the Soquel Demonstration State Forest down to Monterey Bay on the Pacific coast of Northern California. We live in a mixed redwood forest—redwood with pine, cypress, live oak, toyon—on a ridge. Below and away, the forest is dotted with habitation. We can follow the river of Forty-First Avenue as it scythes through the trees and down to the coast. Jill's store is on Forty-First. If she sent up a flare from work, I would see it at the kitchen window.

Hold your right hand in front of you and make a backward C, thumb on the bottom, pointing left. The bay fits in the curve of your hand. The tip of your thumb is Point Pinos Lighthouse in Pacific Grove. The tip of your pointer is the Lighthouse Field in Santa Cruz. Your thumb is Monterey. I live on top of the second knuckle in your pointer. Three windows in my kitchen over the sink frame the entire bay. With binoculars on a clear day, Jill can watch the surfers at Steamer Lane riding in to Cowell Beach by the wharf. The boardwalk roller coasters and amusement rides loop their oddly angled bright colors in their tiny coils.

This is where I cook. On my own recognizance, I am a very humdrum meal provider, but with my meal-prep delivery kits like Blue Apron and Sun Basket, I am a gourmet vegetarian chef. While chopping and dicing, I look south across the water, whitecapped and ruffled, to the Presidio of Monterey and Del Monte Beach. Today is so clear that with a high-powered telescope I could see you walk down Cannery Row to the aquarium. It's hard to believe I can get crabby here, but it happens. Just a decade ago, I was downright depressed in this very kitchen, weeping with my head resting on my folded arms on this same green-and-black granite countertop.

I have to find my way through the noise that old patterns raise.

They spew dread and fear into my brain; I am on edge. Being on edge is okay, but I want to be able to witness it, rather than be overwhelmed by it. Finding a thread or path back to my quiet center requires listening. I listen through the noise in my head. I listen the same way I listen to find the bass note in a piece of music. You discern a tone amid the other tones; it has its own vibration, like a tuning fork humming a certain tone. You could tune a guitar string to the tuning tone.

I have to step out of the kitchen. I go upstairs to my office, where I sit down, center my attention in my body, and breathe. *You are trying to hear what you are telling yourself. What's bothering you today, making you crabby?*

A message is coming up from the depths, not in words but in waves. I put my attention on my breath, detaching it from whatever static or chatter it was tuned to. My mind focuses on my solar plexus, and I take a breath in, then exhale, listening: crabbiness, tight throat. Inhale. Exhale, listening: grief. Inhale. Tears coming on the next exhale. It's grief, really—that's what I want myself to hear. I wrap my arms around my chest, gently holding myself together, feeling fear and loss, feeling alone. A cost of freedom is feeling what you feel.

It's always a clue that I will benefit from listening when something is off. When I am out of tune with someone or myself, or with some commitment of mine, I feel out of sorts. If I listen carefully, I can usually sort out what's bothering me, what's out of harmony and making things feel off. You feel like you're humming when you're in tune. Out of tune is cacophonous.

Intuition works by connecting my attention to some information from my depths, the invisible inner world. It's different from imagination, where you think up scenarios. It's different from ambition, where you look for opportunities. It doesn't come in words. It might come in tears, like it did for me this evening. Or it might come in a glint of attraction, a flicker of humor, or a flash of clarity. You can find the thinnest thread of something and follow it as you pull toward yourself. Like the tingle I got at the seductive slap of a leather glove popping into a mitt. I love that sound; it just makes me look up and pay attention. It doesn't seem like much of a reason to go through the rigors of training, but the thrill is a taproot that drew me in to find more of myself and to discover the many benefits of kickboxing. Sometimes the thread leads to a feeling like anger or sadness; today it is grief. Grief feels like a whole sack of the sad feelings. It feels like cracked deserts. I hear the sound of ice.

The next day, my stem cell donation blood test kit arrives in a medical shipping package. I crack it open and peruse the blood-draw instructions and the examples showing how to label the tubes. You have to fit your name, address, and date, plus the patient's name and ID number, on the little label that wraps around the blood-draw tubes. My hand shakes a little as I fill out a label. I worry: Will it smear? Will my sample get lost? I don't want any room for error. I make an appointment at the local Quest Diagnostics lab to get my blood drawn.

In the morning, I drive to San Jose for my appointment at Quest. At the tiny reception window, I hand the intake nurse the blood-draw package that Kaiser sent me. "I can't use this," she says, and she hands it back to me. "Do you have an order from your doctor?"

"No, I just . . . I just have this request from Kaiser."

"This is not Kaiser."

"No, I know that. I mean, Kaiser sent me the package. I just need blood drawn into these tubes."

"You need an order from your doctor." She holds out the doctor's order.

"This is an order signed by a doctor," I say, taking the sheet back and pointing to the doctor's signature.

"But they didn't give me the right codes." She isn't kidding.

My ob-gyn is in the next suite over. I gather up my stuff and zip out of the waiting room. I jog over to Dr. Kunzel's office and stand at the reception window, looking distraught. Dr. Kunzel's nurse, Sharon, sees me in line.

"What's going on? Are you all right?" she asks, with real interest and no accusation in her tone. Have you noticed that often people are upset that your upset has disturbed their sense of order?

"No. Well, I am, but I need to get this order."

"Order? Let me see." She takes the Kaiser paperwork out of my hand. "Oh, this is for your sister, for the transplant?"

"Yes, how did you remember? Yes." I am so pleased someone is paying attention.

"It was just last month you were in. So, what's the issue?"

"They won't draw the blood without a doctor's order."

"This is an order from a doctor; it's signed here." She points to the signature on the form.

"What can I say? They won't do it because of codes. She said I need an order from my doctor."

"Well, let's get that for you. Just have a seat."

I fold myself into one of those molded plastic chairs with four metal stick legs wearing black rubber feet.

Sharon puts together an order, enters it into the system, and gives me a printout. "Good luck!" she says.

After thanking her in slightly hysterical tones, I jog back to the blood clinic. "Here's the order." I wave it at the receptionist as I burst into the tiny waiting room.

"I'll be right with you," she says, avoiding eye contact. When she reaches out for it, I hand her the order. "Well, I don't have any codes for this."

"You don't have a code to draw blood?"

"No, not just to fill two tubes. You'll have to take it to Kaiser."

"I don't belong to Kaiser. That's an order from Dr. Kunzel, right here in this building."

"I have to have the right codes."

"I'm willing to pay you. It's not an insurance issue, is it?"

"No."

"I'll pay you cash."

"I can't do it."

"But please, my sister is literally dying as we speak. I need to get these samples to Kaiser so I can donate my stem cells!"

"Try Kaiser. But Kaiser in Northern California isn't the same as Southern. So I don't know."

"Please!"

"No."

I go home and call Kaiser and explain that my efforts have been blocked so far. They decide to send me a spittle kit instead. It will be enough to measure the basics. What are the basics? If spittle can do the job, why did they send me two tubes for blood? I want to get the damn tubes filled. I call my next-door neighbor, a registered nurse. She promises to come over after work. "I used to work for Quest; they're totally driven by protocol," she confirms, and she draws the blood for me at home, plunging the needle into a pulsing blue vein in my right forearm and letting it fill first one, then two very neatly labeled little tubes. I FedEx them to the donor testing center the next morning.

For me to cope well with all this, I need to be able to tune in to my inner world and have it guide me. How can you offer a steady arm if your knees are shaking? I'm on an inward journey to my own confidence and ability to be present with whatever happens. The trick is to be available to respond to the whole situation on the spot. You can't do that if your attention and energy are tied up in an unconscious pattern. Your pattern takes over your resources; you can't see anything else.

When I was little, I was terrified to be away from my mother. I mean at ages like seven or ten. My little self just wasn't forming a positive image that could hold me up without someone there to do it. Once, my parents took a trip from our home in Northbrook to California. Daddy was trying to find writing jobs there so we could move. There was some thought that this would alleviate the caustic drinking. We kids were left home with the kindly but hapless Mrs. Burns. For some reason, during her tenure I conceived a distaste for milk; I would consume no milk, cottage cheese, or mayonnaise. Nothing white. I remember committing to resist as a protest against my mother's having abandoned me. I refused to cooperate. No baths, no dinner, no homework. Screaming and fighting, insisting on calling long-distance to California, and no, I will not put my school clothes in the hamper.

Now the universe is talking about taking Linda away on the Long Vacation. There is no one to scream at, no one to refuse. I have to find a stream in my mind that is not controlled by a reactive, unconscious, panicky pattern. One that's not frozen.

BETTER THAN TWINS
Santa Cruz Mountains
Fall 2016

On September 21, at Kaiser, Linda gets her first infusion of R-CHOP. September 29, a mere eight days later, she is admitted to Kaiser with an upper respiratory viral infection, probably pneumonia, and a staphylococcus infection in her heart. She will need five weeks of IV antibiotics to treat the heart infection via a direct PICC line. The first week or so, she stays in the hospital.

On October 6, 2016, Linda calls me from Kaiser. I thought she would die this week. But I also know that results from the HLA test on my blood sample should be coming soon.

When Linda calls, she uses the home line, instead of my cell phone. It has a formality, like this is the phone you use for bad news, when someone dies, or when your stem cells don't match. I expect to hear Linda's husband on the phone with news about Linda. But it's Linda's voice. "Dr. Zhou just called with the results." She sounds so strained, I know it's very bad.

"I'm so sorry, Linda. I tried."

"We're a perfect match," she says. "He said we're like twins, only better. We're a perfect match, ten out of ten."

CHEMO

R-CHOP

Los Angeles
Fall 2016

Like twins, only better, the doctor said. A perfect match. I begin leaping around the house, singing a happy ditty about light shining on me and bursting with relieved joy. We are moving forward with this, the healing is on, everything is coming up roses! We are better than twins, because with my genetics her new immune system will be able to fight any lingering cancer that might arise from her old cells. I hop in my car and drive down to Jill's store on Forty-First Avenue, just to tell her in person. I'm still hopping when I arrive.

But what good will the match do if she dies now from the staph or the pneumonia infection? The hospital is the worst place for an immune-compromised person. The first challenge is for her to heal from those and get back home. Medical interventions can be exhausting. I recall moments during childbirth when I stopped being able to do it. I just let the medical staff take care of it. I faked pushing. I was too depleted. Sometimes the patient just has to let it all go. I think Linda might have gotten to that state.

But Linda is a real force to be reckoned with. She pulls herself right up and out of there. I'm sure a burst of relief-filled energy helps.

It takes five weeks of having antibiotics pumping directly into her veins via the open line, but she's ready to continue the chemotherapy that will beat back the tumors long enough for the transplant to happen. The PICC line is removed, mercifully, and a Port-a-Cath is installed on November 15. The under-the-skin port is much easier and safer. R-CHOP resumes on November 17. That proves so much harder than I imagine. I'm glad we cannot see what lies ahead. It's better to face things as they arrive, with your whole body-mind, than to see them in your imagination, where you cannot really deal with them.

For the next six months, Linda walks through the toxic devastation that R-CHOP brings on. It's really your worst nightmare, because it's endless. You get a shot, and it cooks in you for a few weeks. Just as you're resurfacing from the toxic plunge, you get another shot and plunge again, deeper. Dizziness, nausea, weakness, tiredness intrude into the deepest corners. Sleep is her only respite. "I'm lucky I sleep well. I have no problems with that," Linda says, finding the positive note. She is confined to her home almost entirely over the six months because this chemo obliterates white blood cells, the precursors of immunity components. You are always at risk for what happened to Linda in September—lethal, opportunistic infections. So no dance class, no concerts, no grandchild!

You have to follow all the immune-compromised protocols and stay isolated, and if you go out you have to wear a mask and continually use sanitizer that destroys the skin on your hands. Around the house, you have to keep wiping everything down with alcohol or bleach. The chemo attacks the deformed B cells, but it can't distinguish one fast-growing cell type from another, so there's a hell of a lot of collateral damage. R-CHOP is just lonely and hard and mean. And it builds over time. In Linda's case, it builds over six months.

My Zen friend says he makes an empathic connection with people before a conversation even begins. Then the relationship unfolds inside that connection. I'm not sure what that means. I try to put myself in their shoes. If it were me, I would go squirrelly in the house alone, day after day, with nothing but myself. I might get depressed. I'd likely weep, and I would want to know that people were thinking about me. I would resent being sick. I would be jealous of healthy people. I would want someone to know my suffering and my struggles.

If this were happening to me, what would help me? But can I even imagine? They are living it, and I am only worrying. I'm willing and also afraid to be present with Linda's fear or Rick's loneliness. It seems dangerous to be open to that. Can I risk being more open and vulnerable, let my uncertainty show? Will that be useful in this situation?

I want to be available to Linda if she has feelings like that and wants to use me as an ear. But I don't really know what Rick or Linda might need or feel. I decide it makes more sense for me to deal with my own mind than to guess how to help. Maybe the best help will be a calm mind. Can I drop my fears and defenses and just be here now? I'm willing to do that, I think. I want to show up as a healing presence, whatever it takes. It will probably take kindness. Kindness will be soothing. I need my mother's kindness.

I send cards, little gifts, ginger chews for nausea. I send chicken and beef-bone broth. I know that Linda likes her privacy, and I don't want to pry. I meditate every day before I decide whether to check in, what to ask, or what to say. I want to give her room to express her fears or concerns, her bad mood or whatever. But when I think about it, I can't recall a time when Linda has spontaneously shared her concerns. I think my support means a lot to her, but she never feels the need to reach out, to unload her woes, to ask for courage or a shoulder to cry on. At least not with me. I think it's not Linda's way. Maybe I'm not likely to be the one on whom she depends.

Maybe we are not that kind of friends. Linda has intimate friends, a book club, a dance group. I know her friends visit and check in. I don't know what she might ever need from me, but I intend to be some kind of friend, even silent, if necessary. I ask if Linda wants to learn some game we could play online. She's interested in chess. Ever ready, I take a book on chess out of the library.

I ask how she relates to all the stress from this. "I try to stay in the now," she tells me.

I groan within. I really do not like the "now," as a concept or a place to be. *Why would anyone want to be in the now?* I wonder. *Isn't that where all the stress is happening?* I consider that people must mean something different than this. The now is presumably a refuge from scary or depressing thoughts of the future. But in my view, the scary thoughts *are* what is happening now, and actually I *don't* want to be with them. So how does that work?

Maybe being in the now involves being present with what is present. I guess being present with my scary thoughts is a little better than feeling like I *am* the scary thoughts. When you bear witness, you have to listen to the whole thing, not the story content so much as the feel of it, how it is imprinted in you. What is present? How does it show up in body, emotions, thoughts, sensations? That's not what I really want to do, but Rick and Linda have had the courage to do that. They've looked this dragon in the maw, and they know what's what. I work with being present with what's present when what's present is scary or uncomfortable thoughts and feelings.

Actually, that's useful. I hear the loneliness that I fear; I let it penetrate me and bring its grief. I feel the disbelief. I feel rising anger and resistance like liquid pressure, noticing that it closes my throat and brings a burning sensation. I feel what it is like to feel disconnected, falling through space, alone, really, in an incomprehensible vastness, and I recoil. I witness recoiling. I am here for me as best I can be. A witness to a human being.

You have to set aside time for this stuff. You can't really just stop in the middle of an intersection or on the freeway to be present for an encounter with emptiness or childhood rage. I make sure I meditate regularly to get in my practice hours.

I'm probably overextending myself, because I feel crabby and I get irritated with Linda one morning. I texted, asking how she was doing. Then I was angry that I hadn't heard from her all day. Sometimes I feel like I'm supporting the air. But Linda lets me know that, while she might not show it, my support matters to her.

"Rikki, darling," she texts me in a surprising and rare afternoon plea. "Please don't opt out. I need you in. I do so appreciate everything you do for me. All your suggestions show a lot of thought and research. I certainly don't mean to dismiss them. Sometimes it's easy to interact, but sometimes just returning a text takes so much energy that I don't have. I slept for most of the afternoon, and I'm feeling energetic right now and so I can write this, but I don't always feel this way. But no matter how I feel, I always need you. I am really sorry for offending you this morning."

I feel like an idiot for taking it personally. Then I remember I don't want to feed the feeling of feeling like an idiot anymore.

FIGHT STRATEGY

Mountain View
Fall 2016

Some days are rougher than others. In my monkish life, now retired and free from many distractions, I find that getting to the gym is often the greatest challenge. I get a text from Anh. Anh is a seasoned Muay Thai champion who emigrated from Thailand and is now head coach at my gym. Anh "the Angel" keeps track of his fighters, and, bless my lucky stars, I am one of his fighters.

Anh: "Where you Rikki? You come sparring. Good for you."

Rikki: "I'll be there!"

Anh: "You get here. I hold pads for you."

He keeps me going, he and the people at the gym. I am the oldest gladiator there and, at five foot three, one of the smallest. There are a few women my height, but most folks are taller and bigger boned. Everyone's weight is low, though—these people are honed: flat bellies, swelling shoulders, and muscled thighs. They're also young—mostly under forty. We've built up a group of women who are seriously into sparring. One woman fighting at five foot nine, 120 pounds, has become a Dangerous Person. We are all very proud of her. She has entered several "smoker" fights. A smoker is a light fight between two novices that is not scored but is refereed. No one is trying to hit really hard; they just get the feel of being in a fight. Still, people are hitting and kicking each other, and, like, shit happens.

Anh keeps encouraging me to sign up for a smoker, but I'm scared. I know I would have to train like Floyd Mayweather, and I hate running. It's true, I do hate boring cardio, but I'm also really scared of fighting. So I avoid the smokers. I tell Anh and the crew that I can't risk any injury because I expect to be a donor for my sister. After that, I'll do it, I tell myself and them. My friend Dawn has signed up for the next one, in February 2017.

When I arrive, Anh is doing a private with Benjamin. They're working on combos: jab, cross, front leg kick, teep, two rights. I watch him kick awhile—so tightly executed, all his limbs loose but working together, smooth. Anh glides around the ring, making Benjamin advance. He keeps moving on the balls of his feet, without losing traction. In Muay Thai, you always keep one foot in contact with the ground. That's because you kick in Muay Thai, which is different from boxing. Boxers hop in and out, jump side to side. In Muay Thai you step, because you don't want to get kicked without having some part of your body anchored to the floor. If you're up in the air, you'll get knocked to the ground. Keep that in mind if you're ever in a street fight with a kicker.

Envy helps me get started with jump rope and shadowboxing, and by that time, everyone is starting to arrive. We are amiable and upbeat and ready to beat each other up, like friends should be. "It's only in kickboxing," says my friend Chris, "that you say to someone you just met, 'Oh, that was great. Hit me again!'" You have to admire when someone does get past all your defenses to land a good one. And you appreciate that they pulled back to make a light tap. No one's going for pain or knockouts. It's a sport.

Anh sets the clock, and we start. I look around, spot a guy about six inches taller than I am, and jerk my head up in the universal question *Go a round?* He nods; we take our stance. Move, jab, parry, parry, move. Jab-jab. We start. I forget the combo. I remember—Jab-jab, cross, front leg kick—and I try that. I get bapped after the first jab. I have to remember defense, too! I jab, step out, jab-jab, and feel like I have some control. He moves toward me; I teep. I do it like a push, though, not a snap. Not a good *thunk*; more of a *whoosh*. Lightly, of course. Teeps to the belly can knock the wind out of you and make you feel a little sick. We don't usually do that, but during sparring you get worked up.

I get punched in the nose; I'm angry and rein it in. My energy is up, and I'm looking for an opening: right kick, double. He's distracted, so I move in for an uppercut, but he's moved away. I punch at air and get a hook to the right side of my head for being inside without any cover. I dance away. Now he's rocking toward me with his guard up and I know he's letting me punch awhile. I do my combo and deliver my kick, but he's ready and gets his block up. Just a nice rhythm now—he goes two or three punches and a kick while I keep my guard up; then I go. But then I break the rhythm, trying to get a punch in while he's retracting his fist. I shouldn't—it wrecks the sparring—but I get excited and my body just goes. Anh yells at me to keep control. Sometimes I get angry and start attacking, and it's only discipline that keeps people from hurting me. Bell!

Putting together a decent fight strategy is like developing a mature self-concept. If your fight strategy is based in delusions, you are more likely to get beaten up. If your self-concept is based on a warped or limited view of your human capacity—which you absorbed from your parents' limited understanding—you are more likely to get beaten up. If I think I am smarter than everyone, my arrogance will get me beaten up. If I think I am a victim, people will spot the weakness and take advantage. If I hate myself, I will fail to thrive. A realistic fight strategy for me with most of these sparring partners is to get on the inside, where my shorter arms can connect, but my body is up close, where it is hard to hit me. If I'm getting controlled by a long jab, I need to use my front teep to keep you off me. You want a mature strategy that reflects what is really happening. I get some water and wish the hour were up. Then I see my friend Dawn and I'm excited again. We're about the same height and level of aggression, which is pretty high but dampened by our fear of it. We're both learning as we go. Today we agree to practice blocking kicks. One person throws some strikes and a slow, light kick that gives the other person plenty of warning and time to get up a block. You block by raising your bended knee so your thigh is parallel to the floor, then lock your core and tighten the leg. You want the kicker to get hurt when their shinbone hits your leg. Happily, we never kick that hard, and besides, we're wearing shin guards.

This is how they keep me going while we wait to see what's going to happen with the cancer and the transplant.

CELLS OF HEALING POWER

Santa Cruz Mountains
Winter 2016-2017

While Linda survives chemo, I want to learn everything I can about cells and how I can fabricate cells with healing power. I know that my body is made of trillions of cells, including stem cells. I know that some kind of operational intelligence is active in every cell. A cell is a complete unit of life, carrying out all the functions you might normally associate with a much larger creature, like digestion, procreation, excretion, metabolism, cognition, and mobility. These are conducted in metabolic pathways that manage tremendously intricate biochemical processes. Metabolic pathways are a series of biochemical reactions among cellular components—complex molecules—whose structure contains the instructions on their use.

For instance, the angular construction of water—two oxygen atoms and one hydrogen atom arranged like a V, with the oxygen at the point—creates a tiny separation of charge. The negative goes with the oxygen, the positive with the hydrogen. This separation creates the capacity in a cell to separate different kinds of molecules by their affinity for positive or negative. Charged molecules are attracted or repelled by the charges in water and in each other. Neutral molecules avoid water's polarity and seek each other's company. Cells use this affinity to push and pull molecules in metabolic pathways and to build the tiny organelles that carry out this metabolism. The cell's molecular components "know" how to carry out their tasks because their shapes and charges dictate how they interact with the charges in water and other biomolecules. RNA "knows" how to copy DNA by similar mechanisms. Messenger molecules "know" how to bind to targets. Enzymes "know" how to encourage a reaction. They know without having a mental function; they know by having certain shapes and charges that recognize and interact with other specific shapes and charges. The knowledge is built into their form.

I know that cells are incredibly complex, like a city filled with energetic enterprises. There are factories and farms, cemeteries and libraries. The basic metabolic pathways, such as glycolysis or the electron transport chain, have been preserved despite evolution from the earliest cells to every cell alive today. These metabolic pathways are the family jewels of cellular life on earth. There are sets of chemical reactions that extract and store energy and sets that use the stored energy to build components. For example, there is a chemical pathway that breaks down glucose and captures the energy in a little packet. There is also a chemical pathway for synthesizing glucose, which uses the captured energy stored in little packets. Dozens of metabolic pathways have been passed down, from one living cell to the next, for hundreds of millions of years.

One of the critical components that make possible the living chemistry of a cell is its protective membrane, which controls what goes in and out of the cell. It enables a cell to shield its inner chemical composition and the distribution of shape and charge, so the pathways have a stable environment. The cell membrane is a selective membrane; it allows the passage of specific molecules if they "fit" within one of the channels in the membrane. These channels are created by proteins that make little carriers, rather like boats, to ferry a selected molecule into or out of the cell. Each embedded protein selects a different molecule for passage, as if you had one ferry for Chevy trucks, another ferry for horses, and another for business people. Cells vary the number and kind of ferries—proteins in the membrane—based on conditions. So the membrane becomes a dynamically selective cognitive tool for controlling the intracellular environment and dealing with the extracellular environment.

When cells divide, half of all the material, including all the factories and libraries, goes in each cell. With that material goes all the information about how to grow it and replicate it. After the new cell gets established, it will do exactly that: replicate its internal machinery and grow. Every cell on earth today arose from another cell, going back and back and back to the first successful self-replicating entity. We know of no other way for life to form on this planet, except to come from other life.

A cell, the basic unit of life, like a human, is a continuation of previous life and survives by separating itself from the environment while selectively exchanging information and energy to sustain itself. My life—made of a few trillion cells—is made of the children of previous cells and began when life began, around four billion years ago, not sixty-five years ago. I am not separate from these trillions of cells composing my body, but is my mind separate from them?

Fascinated by the processes in which stem cells specialize into B cells and other blood products, I study the biology of the immune system and B cell functions. I learn how the transplant process works and what my stem cells will have to do. I want to infuse them with my clear intention. I know that sounds a little lunatic-fringe; how can a human mind infuse a bunch of cells with a human-level intention? But that's just how I feel about it. And isn't that a key question William James posed in his 1907 lectures at Harvard? Can a mental state affect the state of matter?

My intentions for myself are focused on stabilizing my mind, befriending myself, and attuning to ways I can support Linda. My intention for my stem cells is that they become power healers. No one understands how holding an intention in your mind affects your body. But every musician, athlete, and dancer in the world believes it does.

And look at it this way: All living systems already exhibit intention at different levels. To intend means "to mean, to plan, to apply with energy, to purpose." Cells intend to, and do, carry out metabolic activities. For example, a cell intends to digest food. For that to happen, a series of complicated and interdependent chemical reactions occurs, including DNA transcription and protein synthesis, and those result in a chunk of food getting engulfed by a protein in the cell membrane and carried across the membrane into the cell. A series of interactions propel the food to a factory where it can be broken down into energy packets and reusable components. This is done auto-dynamically, without an apparent driver, but with a purpose and with energy that result in digestion of food. Similarly, a cell intends to compile proteins, to exchange messages with other cells, and to prepare for mitosis. Each of these activities requires the coordinated action of thousands of components.

Cells are intentional creatures. If they are going to have intention anyway, why not tune that intention with my high-level intention? We are the same person, aren't we? Maybe it's impossible, but how can you know? It feels right to me. I want to infuse my cells with whatever is the cellular translation of "Heal Linda's immune system. Make it strong. Attack any remaining cancer cells, but don't attack any of Linda's healthy host tissues." Be prolific, be active, be smart. I transmit this intention over and over.

Because it is important, and who knows? How do we know how things really work?

We don't. The worlds of matter and of mind are understood to a degree, but at some point our knowledge of both melts into mystery. The contemporary scientific paradigm is based on an information-processing model. Living things are viewed as information processors that take in data in many forms, including light and food, and organize it into us. Living matter is dynamic, creative, entropy creating, yet also mysterious. We know a lot about cellular biology, but we do not know what makes molecules come alive. It's a mystery. Neuroscience shows that thoughts and feelings can be automatically triggered when various stimuli activate certain neural correlates. Experiments show that our sense of "choosing," in some circumstances, appears to occur after our unconscious systems have already put the choice into action. Where is the choice? Where is the chooser? We know a lot about how the brain works, but we don't know how it relates to our awareness and sense of identity. How awareness occurs is a complete mystery.

Within that mystery is something alive that sustains my cells, my awareness, and my sense of identity. Can that aliveness direct a strong intention to my stem cells?

I have to try. Meditation and breathing techniques from several forms of yoga and Buddhism have lead me to transformations and shifts I did not anticipate. If that can surprise me, maybe there's more beneath the covers. I've come to sense that the opaque inner world is very real. It is more than an empty space where thoughts, impulses, or reactions burst out like fireworks in an empty sky. The inner world feels alive, vivid, and gritty. This is where I unbend into forgiveness, reach understanding, sing praises, and grieve losses. There is something alive here, a vitality that seems to embrace and include everything that happens within me. If I block it, it will not come into the world.

I tackle both bodily fitness and mental well-being. Vegan whole-food supplements, blended smoothies, nutritious protein bars, and fruits and nuts go to the gym with me. I get enough sleep. At home, I eat wholesome vegetarian food. (I also eat chocolate, cookies, and ice cream, because I love them.) Meditating daily, I rest in silence and let my sense of self absorb that. I train in Muay Thai three or four times a week. This is not easy; I get tired and crabby, which means I also get sad and weepy. "I'm just absurd," I mutter, holding my hands over my face. "At my age! Other people don't do this to themselves. Who am I trying to impress?" I get scared of the challenge and the confrontation of sparring. *I work so hard*, my mind whines. *I don't have to push myself like this every day.* But I go anyway. Our situation gives me a good reason to follow a tough discipline better than I ever have or will again. And Muay Thai provides friendships that encourage and inspire me. Every time I walk into that gym and see my trainer, Anh the Angel, I get pumped. "Let's get it going, Anh!" I hear myself saying. If I miss a training or sparring session, my phone will ding with a text from him: "Where you Rikki?" No excuse is an excuse.

Cells and I are cognitive creatures with intention. My experience informs me that intention has real force in shaping what happens next. I am holding the intention that my cells will have a powerful effect on another person at the physical level. My cells and I are not different. I'm not somewhere else. The stakes in this gamble are high, and the risk is nothing to me but possible disappointment. I'm taking a leap of faith:

- Viable donor

- Perfect match

- Successful transplant

- Heal

- Kill tumors, and

- No graft versus host (GVH) disease!

SLIPPING THE JAB,
LANDING THE CROSS
Los Angeles
Winter 2016–2017

After she recovers from the staph infection in the heart valve, nothing horrifying happens for Linda, except for the garden-pipe incident. Linda was FaceTiming with her granddaughter Alaia on her phone. "Let me show you the bugs we have in our garden, Alaia." She bent down and pointed the phone at the roots in the dirt, moving slowly, a camera on the hidden life of the garden. Bam! Shin scraped on standing water pipe.

The skin is the only barrier to infection. Linda is several months into chemo. The hidden life of the garden, its flora and fauna, are rushing past her torn tissues into the surrounding fluid, and she has no defenses, not even some measly pawns. Rick flushes the wound, and they call the hotline nurse at Kaiser. "To Emergency immediately!" says the advice nurse. Bundling the leg in clean gauze, they rush over to Kaiser, a few miles away. Professionals clean out the gash. Linda is in luck this time—there is no subsequent infection. Another jab slipped.

Slipping the jab is Rick and Linda's new cancer management

plan. Before we knew we had a 10/10 match, Rick and Linda brought themselves to an acceptance of Linda's death. They did all the legal and financial paperwork, sat down with their children, and went over everything. They set up a Facebook page where Rick could post the bad news when the time came. They were ready for the drama to end in her death. In June 2016, the California End of Life Option Act went into effect. This law enables terminally ill patients to end their lives before their illness inflicts unbearable torment. Linda and Rick discussed with her cancer doctor the possibility that they would need the prescription that would end her life. They learned that Kaiser and her doctor would support her if it came to that. Can you see yourself having this conversation? For them, death was a real possibility, even a likelihood. But now they're on a new trajectory with each other. There's good reason to expect a future. It's empowering and enlivening for them. It's that vitality, that energy, that you want to tap.

As long as I am alive, I want to access that sense of vitality you need to slip a jab and follow with the right cross. I am realizing as we go through this that my own aliveness has been stifled. I'm inspired to keep shaking myself out of complacency. I want to feel and own my own life's power. How does that get blocked off? Why would you ever *not* feel your own liveliness?

Yet I have known years of depression when my vitality was stopped. I guess there have been a gazillion moments when my life force was tangled in confusion or anxiety. I suspect all that disquiet was the debris of having a fractured self-concept, of thrashing around and not knowing how to settle into my own skin. The key to my empowerment now is willingness to give up stories that keep my self-concept twisted. I can no longer afford to be a twisted sister. I am ready to be the holistic version of Warrior Rikki.

Linda can't be in the Women's March in January 2017, but she can knit. She knits seventeen pink pussy hats that march in Dallas, Washington, and Los Angeles, plus one in a Seattle preschool. Since the 2016 election, like everyone I encounter online or in life, I've been trying to understand what's happening among Americans. We all want our power in these populist times. So many people are outraged, for different reasons. Unsatisfied and often desperate people in disparate situations insist that governments and societies protect our conflicting values and social identities. The struggle for control could hardly be more polarized. The 2016 elections hit like a teep to the national solar plexus, knocking the air out of us and leaving us stunned. Right- and left-wing populism has got everyone's attention. Some social norms that held scary passions in check have crumbled; the press says we have lost the guardrails. Rules will be broken. Sacred cows will be roped. People want power. Voters are fed up with the program.

The liberal view I grew up with held that when the material quality of life improves, people improve. They become more able to deal with life's vicissitudes, more able to thrive, more considerate of their fellows, and more able to grapple with the mysteries of their own being. But I wonder if material improvements really help develop skillful means and attitudes. What seems missing is improvement of our relationship with our own minds and ways to access our own vitality. Consumption does not really satisfy us. We want to enjoy our life force; we want our subjectivity and creativity to matter. We want to feel the joy of our own hearts beating in our own chests.

That call resonates with me. I want to feel the power of my life and vitality. I want to feel the stream of life that is my own self. Have I been suppressing my well-being to get along with the broken world? Now that I can slip a jab, can I follow up with a cross, deliver my own punch? I want to feel the joy of my own heart beating in my chest. I want to be able to say no. To choose. To love more freely. To speak my mind and share my passion. To heal my rootlines.

TRIALS

DONATION TIME!

Los Angeles
March 2017

November, December, January, February—the months of chemo drag on. Linda's Prius memorizes the path from her home to Kaiser, where she goes weekly for infusions or follow-up tests. She's had a few emergency trips to manage potential infections, but she's pulled through—no eye infection, no wounds, no organ failures, though her lungs and kidneys are strained. Finally, it is March 2017: time for the transplant. We are ready to begin the next phase of healing.

Monday. I drive down through the Central Valley of California to stay at Linda and Rick's home in Los Angeles. My part of California is cooler and more moist than theirs, but even they had floods during our El Niño last year, in 2016. California may be able to pull out of drought. We got real rain that year, adding depth to the snowpack that feeds our rivers and reservoirs. I drive past a full San Luis Reservoir at the east end of the Pacheco Pass, and I see water in the viaduct that crosses Interstate 5. There is reason to hope.

My role in the family has become Warrior Rikki, someone who has achieved epic status already. Warrior Rikki is conceived as a kind of modern samurai. I meditate, engage in martial arts combat, eat gourmet vegetarian meals, and read haiku. Everyone believes Warrior Rikki's stem cells will be vigorous, youthful, potent, compassionate, and successful. We share a black-and-white headshot of me with flexed fist that shows off my best ruffian side. Sweat drips through my plastered hair, and a solid look of resolve and strength fills out my features. My shoulder muscles leap out. A myth has grown up about this Warrior Rikki's stem cells saving the day. My family likes this image to focus their aspirations. I'm a little embarrassed, but this is the part I am to play, so Warrior Rikki becomes Rikki Stormborn, Mother of Cells. I am tough and lean and resolute. Linda tells her cancer doctors, "Have you met my sister? She is a force to be reckoned with." I shake my fist and make an indomitable, though soft, roaring sound. *I got this*, the gesture says.

I have come a long way from Troublemaker Rikki, who escaped from the local Catholic school after fifth grade like a wild hooligan but never really had bad intentions.

March 1960

Billy Wilkie had a close-cut, military-style haircut, so there was nothing for me to grab after he swung and missed. I had to throw my arm around his neck and try to get him in a half nelson. A half nelson, my dad taught me, was one of the ways you can hold somebody by the neck and still have a hand free so they can't mess with you. Billy Wilkie had some kind of mental problem from being adopted, like he felt crappy all the time and started fights. I understood Billy, so we were kind of friends, so we fought sometimes.

Father Sullivan broke up the fight and sent us in early from recess to sit at our desks and pout like good children. Usually I didn't mind; I was happy to read a book, and I had been racing through *The Hidden Harbor Mystery*. But I was angry today because Old Lady Crowe had taken away my science experiment.

I brought a scientific project to my fourth-grade class with Miss Crowe. I discovered how electricity flows with a simple battery, wires, a switch, a socket, and a light bulb. The diagram was in one of the books in Daddy's library, and I had Mommy drive me down to the Woolworth's in town, where you could get everything. I just needed the socket. I found a switch in the garage, and some wires. Daddy had these big, tall six-volt batteries for a lantern or something. All I had to do was run the wires from the battery to the switch, switch to socket, and back again through the switch! I turned that light on and off with awe and respect for hours. I loved that little thing. There really was something flowing around the wires, and you really could shut it on and off.

So I brought it in to show off. But Miss Crowe Face was mad at me for playing with it during class, so she took it away from me. And that was just not fair. So when the class came back in from recess, I thought I would demonstrate to them how Miss Crowe Face behaved.

We sat in alphabetical order in neat rows, and my last name is West, so I was in the back of the room. After everyone returned from recess and Miss Crowe turned to the blackboard, I quietly stood up and began my pantomime imitation of Miss Crowe scolding the innocents sitting next to me. One hand on my hip, the other wagging forcefully, I shook my head and mouthed the famous, "You will not get away with that in my class, young lady. If I see that again, it's off to Mother Superior with you!" Kids near me started to laugh. I sat down, but not quickly enough. It was off to Mother Superior with me.

You had to walk down a red stripe on the edge of the linoleum when you walked in the halls at St. Norbert's. The joy of stepping off that line was worth the inevitable ruler thwack on the hand or rap on the side of the head. But what I hated was how guilty I knew Mommy would make me feel for getting in trouble again. I wanted Daddy to come pick me up and get me out of there.

And this time, he did. And Daddy was so mad at them for taking away my light that Mother Superior had to give it back and he said he did not have to spend his money at that institution anymore. Which was almost true; he finished paying that year's tuition, but the following September, I was "free free free" at Crestwood Middle School in Northbrook, Illinois. I wanted to be like Daddy when I grew up, so I wouldn't have to put up with stuff or spend my money at that institution.

We will do the stem cell donation at City of Hope in Duarte. A century ago, Duarte was a citrus farming community, maintaining a tuberculosis sanitarium on acres where City of Hope grew up. Now Duarte is largely a bedroom community for its residents and a world-renowned healing center for its patients. The drive to and from City of Hope is about an hour and a quarter, sometimes more in traffic. There is always traffic on some part of the route. We can take the 405 to the 101 if the interchange is not totally stopped, or we can get to the 210 via the 10 and the 605. We take the 101 route. The trick is, on the way there, stay to the left. The freeways and naming systems change and re-change, and you can never be sure the name of the highway you're on. But if I stay to the left, Google maps could call it the "Glendale Freeway" while the sign says Pasadena, and I'll still be fine. I don't have to worry about that this trip. Rick will drive me to and from the donation center and stay with me all day.

I bunk in Ari's old room, which becomes Alaia's room when she visits. Ari is now a mathematics teacher at Santa Monica High School. His signed poster of the Minnesota Twins is still pinned to the wall. Linda's daughter, Lise, left a rectangular yellow-and-red Tibetan *zafu*, about eight inches high, that will work perfectly for my daily sitting. I find Alaia's tiny pink-striped socks and star-spangled pull-ups in the dresser drawer. On the dresser stands a three-by-five-inch framed photograph of our old house in Northbrook. It looks ominous in

black and white, like a shot of Bates Motel. Maybe I'm just in a grim
mood.

Tuesday. I wake early, around 5:30 a.m. It is cold in their house.
Despite being in Los Angeles, they live in a corridor that brings a
breeze straight in from the beach, just a few miles away. It keeps the
air cool and fresh around their home, especially in spring. I've never
been one to meditate happily in the cold. I haven't the discipline.

I wrap myself in a blanket and bumble out to the kitchen to get
coffee. I'm the first one up. Linda claims they can't hear the coffee
grinder, so I go ahead and grind a cup's worth. Using the single-cup
drip filter, I prepare a cup, take it back to my *zafu*, settle on my
crossed legs, and get toasty enough to fall asleep. Instead, I open my
journal and write out my intentions. I write out my aspiration. The
physical act of writing slows my thoughts down. I remember what I
am doing. Then I finish my coffee and meditate.

Today I have to get my health checked at Kaiser, where I will be
admitted as a temporary patient whose medical costs will be billed
to Linda's medical insurance. This causes enormous confusion, but
there actually is a protocol for handling it. Tomorrow I will be referred
and admitted to City of Hope to get testing done there also. Kaiser
has a working relationship with City of Hope and refers patients to
that hospital's services, just as it is doing with Linda. Doctors from
Kaiser go on tour of duty at City of Hope. It's one wonderful healing
family held together by nurses, as far as we can tell. Said nurses take
tubes and tubes of my blood, measure my pulse and blood pressure,
listen to my heart, x-ray my chest, and ask me to fill out quantities of
forms. I write happily, confident we are closing in on this.

Tomorrow at City of Hope I will also get trained in how to deliver
shots. I will administer shots of Neupogen into my belly for a few
days prior to harvest. This stuff stimulates the production of the pluripotent stem cells that I am donating. When your body produces
more stem cells than you need, they get pushed out of your bone

marrow into your bloodstream. There, they last a few days or so, then die out and get expelled in urine. My body's job is to produce and push into my blood an extra 4.5 million stem cells per kilogram of Linda's body weight. I will nourish these cells with daily doses of vegan whole food, vitamins, and protein powder spun up in a blender with fresh fruit. I'm pretty sure we're in Fat City.

Wednesday. The three of us make it to City of Hope parking lot by 9:00 a.m., despite all traffic odds. Rick goes with Linda to her appointments, and we'll meet up later. We both have blood labs to do. I get weighed, measured, and de-blooded. I fill out forms with a Bic ballpoint pen and wonder briefly when these were manufactured. I balance on a plastic chair next to a tongue of table with an armrest for blood withdrawal. Only half-sheltered behind a shower curtain ringed to a curved aluminum rod about a foot above my head, I am waiting for the Neupogen trainer.

A nurse looks from her desk so suddenly it catches my eye. She stands up, clipboard in her right hand while her left flips a few pages back, checks something, then folds the top three sheets back so the fourth is exposed. She steps out from her desk and walks over to me.

"Mrs. West?"

"Ms. Yes."

"You went to Mexico in January?"

"Pardon me?" I stammer. "Mexico? No . . ."

"It says you got off a cruise boat in Cozumel?" she asks, tone uplifting, as baffled as I am.

"Oh, yes, at the wharf, yes. We just walked around. I didn't eat anything. What's the question?"

"It's the Zika virus"—as if this explains something to me.

I can hear the clacking of a keyboard over the murmur of voices coming from the television set tuned to CNN in the adjacent waiting room. My nostrils can just catch the irritation of hand sanitizer in the air. My eyes are looking at her face while everything slows down. I can no longer see the hospital green of someone's scrubs in my peripheral vision. "Maybe just ice cream," I say stupidly. I can feel the skin on my face sagging down toward my teeth. I squint to get everything back up where it belongs.

"We have a restriction against donors who have traveled to places with Zika," she says.

Jill and I went on a cruise the previous January with friends of ours from Florida. I had rather forgotten about it until I was filling out the forms. We met up with our buddies on the ship and sailed gaily out to the Caymans, around Cuba, and into port at Cozumel on the way home. I got off for an ice cream, or a walk around on land.

"Oh my god." The blood flows out of my face and throat, plummeting to my belly. Adrenaline whirls through me, making my heart change rhythm and my mind shut down. "No. Wait."

"But you stayed in port?" she asks, clarifying, still hopeful. I really have stopped breathing. Was she actually saying I couldn't be a donor because of the Zika virus? *That can't be what happens in this story,* I think. Zika virus is not going to become an obstacle, no way.

"Yes," I manage. "I was just off the ship a few hours."

"Let me check. I think that's all right."

She is gone for a long, long time; maybe minutes. I wait impatiently, doing breathing exercises to calm down so I can think. They have tests to determine whether you've been exposed to Zika, right? Could I be carrying the virus without having developed an infection? Is that even possible? My skinny butt hurts from pressing on the plastic seat. My back is starting to sag. Finally, I can wait no longer. I get up from my station where they took my blood and left me to worry endlessly. I don't want to barge into any other spaces, but I want to find that nurse.

"Can I help you, dear?" comes immediately from a nurse working on files at a table stand nearby.

"Yes. I'm waiting for the Neupogen nurse, but really I wanted to know what they said about the Zika exposure."

She shuffles the charts on her table and finds mine. "I think . . . Let me check. Is that what you're waiting for?"

"Yes. No, the Neupogen. But she was going to find out . . ."

"Let me find Alice about that, and I'll call Stella about the Neupogen. You need the demo, right? How to give your shots?" She wears a flowered light jacket over her blue scrubs, and the name pinned above the pocket is Irna.

"Thank you, Irna."

She's off, but not for long—within a few moments, she comes back around the corner. "You're fine with the Zika thing. It's no problem if you stayed in port and it's been a few months. Let me just get a volunteer to walk you over to meet Stella for the training demonstration."

"It's okay, then? I can still donate?"

"Yes, no worries, dear." She smiles and touches my arm as she takes out her phone.

Stella gives me a crash course in how to administer the shots, and then I'm finished with City of Hope for today. I meet up with Rick and Linda in one of the waiting rooms. Eventually, we navigate ourselves across the Southern California highway system to Kaiser Cadillac pharmacy to get the shot kits and take care of all that so I'll be ready to start the shots in the morning. Linda has gotten these injections dozens of times to urge her WBC up to survival levels, but never more than one a week. In my body, the dosage will stimulate superproduction. Over the next couple of days, my lymph nodes swell up with white blood cells and pluripotent stem cells, piling up like stacks of hay before the harvest.

LISTENING
Los Angeles
March 2017

Thursday. Supporting people who are going through something this prolonged and dramatic is not straightforward. They are facing a radical, permanent, and sudden change in their life trajectory and life story. They have so much to absorb and so many feelings that must come along with it. How can you show up for people existing with that kind of intensity, that kind of life-in-your-face situation, without being annoying? Wouldn't anything you say be irritating just because you don't have to deal with this?

This week at Linda's house, I hold back from talking a lot or trying to be clever. I try to be still. I work to manage my own agitation and not to fuss over others just to comfort myself. This involves a lot of noticing and breathing. Then again, people need to connect with other real people. Wouldn't they want to feel that someone could at least see them and someone at least cared? Maybe I'm too aloof. Maybe I should be more talkative. No, maybe I should . . . I don't know. I meditate in the morning and sometimes during the day on Lise's red-and-yellow Tibetan *zafu*.

—

I try to drop all that and just relax, to be simple and genuine. You can't plan simple and genuine, but you can notice when you're not. I slowly calm down into the situation without giving in to a need to fix things. I want to be kind but honest, though not heavy. Present and relaxed, but not annoying. Plus, I have fears and grief to manage. I try to listen to intuition without getting flooded by my own confusion.

We set up the Neupogen kit in the kitchen. We wipe down the kitchen table surface with an alcohol wipe, which seems like overkill. Then I swab an area in the inner circle on my belly with alcohol. I will be shooting a pattern of concentric circles around my belly button over the next few days. Taking out a Neupogen packet, I peel the foil back and remove a tiny syringe with the prepackaged medication. I remove the plastic needle cover and set it on the table. Now I just need to pinch my sanitized skin and plunge the needle while depressing the piston. Done. I whip out the needle. No pain and no blood. Taking out a second packet, I repeat the steps, puncturing a spot about an inch away from the first and on the same circle. This is easy. We gather up the foil and plastic packaging and toss everything in a plastic bag. I won't feel anything for two days; then my lymph nodes will start to swell up, as they do when you get sick and your immune system makes a lot of white blood cells. I'll be making so many stem cells, they'll be maturing into white blood cells that load up the lymph nodes and spill, along with millions of stem cells, into my bloodstream.

Later in the warm spring afternoon, we go outside to get some air in the backyard. Linda doesn't go in her swimming pool today. She snuggles into one of the padded chairs around the round outdoor glass table sitting under the pergola. She stays wrapped in the warmth of a shawl over her jeans and sweater. She has a book, but it has been hard for her to concentrate lately. I wonder if she even knows her name, given what she's endured. I ease my feet and legs beneath the surface of the water. It feels silky and pleasant against my skin. This family discovered how wonderful it is to have a pool when Alaia, Linda's granddaughter, learned to swim. Suddenly everyone loves hanging around by the pool. But today, Rick went to the gym and Linda will soon fall asleep. I lie on a pair of foam noodles and look through my Maui Jim prescriptions for birds in the passion fruit and trumpet vines that climb the backyard fences, a blue Golden State Warriors cap protecting my eyes from the glare.

BOUNDARIES
Los Angeles
March 2017

Friday. I take Santa Monica Boulevard over to Sepulveda to the A4 Fitness boxing club. I'm doing a one-on-one with coach Achim.

"Every strike, make it from your core." Achim twists his whole torso when he demonstrates the left hook. Hip, waist, chest, shoulder, and the attached arm move as a unit. Bam-bam-bam. "Arm parallel to the floor."

Most people let their elbow drop when executing a hook, but just think about it: All the power is coming from the turn in the hip being carried straight through via your forearm. Letting the elbow drop destroys the delivery of power to the target.

"It's in the footwork."

I stare at his feet. I thought it was in the hips! Even on the jab, he has a slight twist in the rear foot that puts some momentum from the rear leg into the power train. I try to copy that.

"Don't punch with your arms like that." He demos flopping arms that could be slapping someone with a damp dish towel. "Punch with your core." I tighten up the abs so I look more like him. "Keep your hands loose; throw with your core and shoulder." I work this for a while.

"Use the teep to keep me off you," Achim says, coming at me with jab-jab, cross. Jab-jab, cross. The teep is a front-facing push kick. You can do it with the front or the rear leg, but the front leg is most common. You use it like a jab in boxing. "Be strong." He clenches his body to show me what strong looks like. "Hold your body strong, raise your leg, and make a hard stop on me."

I sidestep, see the jab coming, quickly stick my left foot in his belly.

"Not pushing. Make a hard line. Say, 'Stop. Stop.'"

He wants my knee to come up and my foot to shoot out fast and connect right where I want to stop him. My teep is my boundary maker. Here comes the jab; I teep. Jab, teep. Jab, teep.

"Make your rear leg stronger. Keep me off you. Say no. Make me stop."

I work my leg but can tell the extra power I need comes from the core. The stopping power comes from the rear leg and torso, right through the rigid core. Or it flops out in a flabby core.

I want to learn this maneuver. It takes strength and balance and power in the legs, but what I want is the power in the center of me to say, *No!* I want to feel that energy come up and set a no-cross line that I own and I create with my own power. When he teaches me this, I can't help but notice that this physical act makes me joyful. Teeping is fun. When someone is coming at you, and you can bop them right there while you stay balanced and ready, and they go off balance and look hurt and surprised, it feels great. You naturally want to follow up with a cross, hook, and rear body kick.

It's liberating! I think. *You can control your own space.* Thoughts come and go quickly in class. You have to get back to your body right away. I store this to think about later.

We set up to do some combos. Working in pairs, one person holds the pads while the other does the combo. I get the pads and hold for a jab-jab, cross, left low kick. My partner is light on his feet, dancing with the punches, getting his weight behind him but keeping the tap light enough that I can handle it in the pad. You have to hold firmly and slap back against the hit or kick just a little bit. You don't want the pad to recoil into your face—it leaves a nasty discolored lip. When it's my turn to strike, I deplete myself slamming the damn pads. Bat-bat-bam-boom. Bat-bat-bam-boom. You get into your own rhythm. It's the most natural thing in the world. It's all yours. In sparring, your opponent will use it against you, throwing it off by striking between beats. You have to learn to balance your weight and hold your own when your opponent tries to mess you up. But first you need to learn what is your own. You have to get to know what really works for you so you can try to establish that at the beginning of a session.

When you extend for the jab, your weight is all forward and to the left. So you sit down in the punch and keep your weight centered, with your hips under you like a cup, holding your upper body. Now the punch is coming from the rear leg, through the hip, into the shoulder. The gloved fist is just the knot at the end of the whip. Whhhiip! Whhhiip! That's how a jab should shoot out if you are using it to hurt or distract. I am learning my strength, and we are all surprised by it. Even an old lady can be a weapon. It's all about composure, balance, and owning your space.

Driving back to Linda's, I'm really jazzed about developing a strong teep. I see how to use it more effectively now. Setting a boundary, having the right and even the power to set a boundary, to tell another person, "No, that's my space," seems like a radical act, even a political one. Have I been unwilling to claim my own space? Did I really not learn how to set boundaries in my family of origin? Why does teeping feel like a superpower?

PHOTOGRAPHS
Los Angeles
March 2017

Saturday. Rick makes a pot of coffee every morning; it is a comforting routine. The coffee grinder and thermos-drip apparatus stand in their place on the countertop near the breadboards. He pours beans from a ceramic jar into the grinder cup and slides the container into place beneath it. The fruity, smoky scent fills the air as the whir of the grinder stops. He puts the grounds into the coffee filter and pours hot water into the upper chamber. Soon a strong cup with a dash of cream is in my hand. We've got the *LA Times* and our iPads to read the news. I don't talk about the articles I read. I am being very quiet, very Zen, committed to being of service without being annoying without abandoning myself while being present and available. . . . I'm clearly too busy to talk.

Morning light flows over the gardenia window box, through the wooden shutters, onto the big, round wooden table. It was at this very kitchen table just a few years ago that I argued so earnestly with Mom about her physical care. Hank had endured a serious and massive heart attack. I helped take care of Mom at Linda's home, near Hank in the hospital, since Linda was in Chicago. When Hank got out of the hospital, he came to Linda's and was resting there with Mom before heading back home in the morning.

September 2012

"Mom," I pleaded, "you and Hank need more help. He can't do everything alone. You've got to move down here, closer to people who can assist you guys."

Linda lives in a pleasant old West LA neighborhood of well-tended bungalows and new mansions. Elizabeth lives in an adjacent neighborhood. They can drive to everything they need, even a Kaiser hospital, within a few miles. Though LA traffic strangles efforts to go farther, within the neighborhood and linked neighborhoods they have easy freedom. If Mom and Hank could get into a condo in a neighborhood where Linda and Bethy could reach them, it could really upscale the quality of their days. And we'd get Mom back into our lives.

But the stubbornness of early dementia had set its teeth on this one.

"You fucking bitch," Mom growled at me. "I'm not leaving my home. Don't speak another word to me. Hank, get me out of here."

That scared me! I had never heard that shocking sound before, the sound of her malice and gravelly anger. My mother was a gentle soul, usually attentive and mostly kind. Yet was this voice completely unknown? It rankled the back of my mind until I found the thread. It sounded like the same cruel taunting that incited my father's drunken rage decades ago. You could hear them downstairs if you sat in the hallway and waited. Sometimes you had to sit on the stairs because the monsters were active and might get you in bed. So you had to get up and sit on the stairs, away from the dark closet and out of reach of anything under the bed. There, you could rest safely if you didn't lean against the walls, from which dark arms with long, sinister fingers might extend to squeeze the life from your neck. From this tiny perch, I could sometimes hear the sick, confused voices of resentment and anger discharging between them. They were dark, upside-down sounds of my loving family spewing into space. I was so lonely.

My whole system seized up with grief and rage when Mom snarled at me in Linda's kitchen. I couldn't speak. I felt orange and red inside. It wasn't so much being called a bitch as it was the total wall that came down between us. That wasn't my mother—yet it was. Her voice triggered the kind of panic I felt on the stairs as a child.

I stood in the middle of the kitchen. "I have to go home," I said. I turned and went to my bedroom to pack my bag. Two minutes later I walked right through the dining room and the kitchen and out the door. I fled. My whole intention had been to continue supporting them until Hank was well enough to drive them home, probably in the morning. But I packed my bags and left within minutes. I wept for most of the six-hour drive back to the Santa Cruz Mountains.

Now I'm standing in that same kitchen, its L-shaped countertop extending into a breakfast nook holding the wooden table made for them by Rick's Uncle Jack, remembering. The refrigerator is covered with over forty years' worth of family photographs, narrating events and highlights with the people who fill their lives. There are stories here of friendship and loss, betrayal and hope. My own refrigerator is a blank stainless-steel wall, but Linda surrounds herself with the people who gave or begged forgiveness, patience, endurance, and love, who brought joy and heartbreak. Daddy is usually not on the refrigerator. There aren't any recent pictures of him. He died decades ago, when Linda's adult children were just children.

Linda and Bethy took care of him then. He was homeless when he got sick with lung cancer, and they had to find a place for him at

Veterans. We grieved his death, but, as Elizabeth said, it fulfilled his lifelong dream. He actually asked me to help him die once. In high school I knew people who sold drugs on campus, just one or two pills that they probably stole from a parent's medicine chest. But Daddy wanted enough to die from. He asked me to get them for him. He had returned from a writing trip to Florida, where, I thought, he had written material for Dom DeLuise, or perhaps it was the Smothers Brothers. These guys were very successful comedians at the time. Maybe things went poorly. He had locked himself in his study for a couple of weeks. I don't know if he was eating; I was supposed to be studying chemistry. He told me one day that he had to die; could I get him some pills? I just said okay. Linda heard me on the phone, calling friends, asking who had reds. She put the kibosh on the whole deal. What if she hadn't stopped me? This is the kind of thing that happened around my father. Razors and shotguns had to be kept away from him.

The chemo is damaging Linda's lungs, and the effects right now are particularly acute. It's hard for her to walk around. Her hair is all gone, and she stays warm under a scarf. I'm scheduled to do some Muay Thai in the afternoon.

DONATION

City of Hope, Duarte
March 2017

Monday. Donation Day.

Rick chops on the cutting board set atop the tile countertop, as light from the window streams in above the sink. He's dicing the fruit for their breakfast cereal. I don't want to eat because I'm nervous about needing a bowel movement during the procedure. "Oh, your body will realize it just has to wait. Don't worry," Linda tells me. She's been through so many procedures, she speaks from the best kind of knowledge: direct experience. I decline food anyway. Perhaps I'm a little nervous.

"Alexa, play KUSC," Rick says, and she does. A lively string piece, a minuet or dance of some kind, jingles through the kitchen. I pack light snacks and drinks. Rick will eat lunch at the cafeteria on the City of Hope campus. He is taking me to the infusion center and will hang out with me all day. "Alexa, volume up," says Rick. The Great Composer Quiz comes on, asking something like, "Which conductor always wears a white carnation when conducting?" and Rick says, "Sargent." "Alexa, volume down," Linda says.

After breakfast, the two of us load ourselves into Linda's forest green Prius. Linda and I have identical cars, different years, although that was not intentional. We just happened to pick the same model and color of hybrid Toyota. We are different in many fundamental ways, but we also had a secret language and just passed an identical-twin HLA test.

Rick bobs and weaves up the 405 onto the 101 and stays to the left until we are decanted into the Brawerman Center at City of Hope. I'm prepared for a prolific session in the donor throne over the next six or seven hours. There's a porta-potty next to the bed under the window. We're on the second floor, so I'll be able to squat down without inviting curious onlookers. They're going to stick one needle in my right arm and draw my blood through a tube into a machine. The machine contains a centrifuge and all its accoutrements, which will techno-magically spin down each blood sample to isolate the layer with the stem cells and extract them. The rest of my blood is remixed and returned through a vein in my left arm. My lymph nodes are swollen; I'm bursting with stem cells. They've scheduled two sessions for me, since I'm old and slight of build—one today and one tomorrow.

I set out all my stuff on the bed trays so all is within easy reach. I've brought some fruit, nuts, a protein bar made with almonds and honey, and sixty ounces of water. I've got my Kindle for reading, and, if I want, I have some audiobooks on my phone and movies on my iPad.

My dedicated nurse, Sarah, tests my blood vessels and finds the right spot on each side. She implants the needles, then screws the collection and return tubes onto them. I am hooked up to the harvester. It's painless, like donating blood. The collection bag is hanging from a hook jutting out from my IV stand, looking every bit like a simple blood-collection bag.

Rick goes out for a walk and a visit to the library. I drink half a gallon of water to combat dehydration that could occur from removal of my blood. The biggest challenge we have is managing all the tubes and wires when I have to step out of bed to the porta-potty. I nibble my snacks and read, and after a few hours, Sarah holds out the bag. "Looking good!" she says. Sure enough, it is beginning to accumulate a dark fluid.

"Are those stem cells?" I ask.

"Yep. Just collecting here in this bag."

"And then what do you do to freeze them?"

"We just freeze the bag."

"Let's get a photo," I say, and I send it out via text message to the family. I'm so jazzed, I look like I'm running a marathon, eyes energized and smile shining.

In two more hours, I am a hero, or at least I've completed a hero's challenges. They remove the needles and tape me up. I gather all my things, and they load me into a wheelchair. Rick escorts me down to the exit, where I get up and walk to the car. I feel great, not weak at all.

In the evening, the attending nurse calls me at Linda's and tells me I've produced 6.5 million cells per kilogram of Linda. Nearly 50 percent more than required. We are in Fat City indeed. I stay at Linda and Rick's to recover a few days before I drive home.

DELAY
Los Angeles
March 2017

Wednesday. We are taking things slowly, reading in our rooms. Reading is the family pastime. We all read several books a month, and I always thought it was Daddy who set the reading standard. But now I cannot picture him sitting down with a book the way I can picture Mom. I think he was too antsy to read much. I can more readily picture him hunched over his old black Underwood, Parliament clamped between his teeth. In my memory, white cigarette smoke curls around him and his laughter exhales from it like a warning. He sort of chortles at the paper as he punches keys with two reinforced fingers.

Linda likes to spend some daytime hours in Lise's old room, later a hobby room, now a guest room. It's light and feminine and fluffy. East-facing windows let the morning light filter through the blinds. She might have a little sniffle. We are terrified of little sniffles now.

The seven-cycle R-CHOP ordeal is over, and the stem cells are harvested, but we have not started the transplant process. We await results from a PET scan to determine the condition of the tumor. She knows the tumor has shrunk; she could feel the relief in pain and pressure months ago, after the first chemo round. We wanted it dead, but, recalcitrant to the point of non-responsiveness, it might live on. A little bit of live tumor would be all right. Since Linda is getting a stem cell transplant, all her new immune system cells will have the new genetics. They will see the tumor cells as alien and mount a defense to destroy them. In fact, if any of Linda's original stem cells survive the transplant to produce cancerous cells, they'll be attacked as aliens also.

Thursday. We feel like we should feel like celebrating. Rick's mother has been asking Linda when she will be well enough to socialize. Ruth would really like to solemnize Linda's progress by going out to dinner. That is her favorite way to observe love and gratitude. Ruth is ancient. She has survived two husbands, cancer, and a severe stroke. She has a way of demanding arrangements that leaves Rick nearly helpless. She is the opposite of my mother in that way, as an outward pressure. My mother was more of an inward pressure.

Ruth invites us all out to dinner at the Grill on the Alley, a special feast for traditional LA diners.

"No," I cry, "don't go! It's a hotbed of germs. All those people, touching the chairs, the tabletops." Why do we go? We pick Ruth up at her apartment, and Rick drives us to the Grill. We are seated immediately around an old-fashioned, heavy wooden table laid with big silver cutlery and large white linen napkins. Brass and mirrors reflect the gleam of polished wood. I can smell charring steak and roasting meat.

Ari joins us at the restaurant. Linda's head is protected in a cloth rolled-brim cloche the color of ivory. We are all upbeat, saying how sure we are that Linda will be fine. But a transplant is hard, and Linda is beaten up from chemo. If only she could have a rest. Instead, we are in a public place, a real danger zone. The cutlery is not wiped down, the doors are not wiped down, the dishes are not wiped down. Twice, Linda pulls a small container of sanitizer from her bag and squishes a few droplets onto her fingers. The waiter is bringing bread, condiments, glasses that have been god knows where. Now, salt and pepper shakers appear on the table. Linda picks up her menu. The pan-fried Dover sole is renowned, and I think everyone who is not vegetarian orders it. I order a salad and an eighteen-dollar plate of grilled asparagus. We are awash in germs; bacteria lurk on every surface; there are viruses on everything. Trillions of viruses, strands and strands—how can you avoid them?

Friday. The PET results are in. Linda and Rick go in to see Dr. Zhou, who is Linda's transplant doctor at City of Hope, which I have begun to call Cope. The PET shows some live tumor, but that's apparently within the plan. The expectation is that the new immune system, built on my genetics, will find and kill this bit of tumor after the transplant. Just one more test, scheduled at Kaiser on a Friday evening. We're on a tight schedule. As soon as the last chemo dose fades, the tumor will kick-start new growth.

Around 6:30 p.m., Linda and I drive over to Kaiser for the test. Things are quiet in our department, and we wait only a few minutes for the nurse. Linda gets the scan, and things might still have worked out just fine if we didn't walk out through the emergency room, a shortcut to our car, which is filled on Friday night with patients suffering influenza virus, rhinovirus, and adenovirus—ordinary, abundant, infinitesimal threads of single- or sometimes double-stranded ribonucleic acid. But we do walk out that way. So between the Grill and the emergency room, exposure is hardly avoidable.

Saturday. Things are suddenly not jim-dandy. One of the damn strands of virus from somewhere has landed in Linda's nasal passages and is invading her cells left and right. With her deformed B cells and the havoc of chemo, she has a super-low white blood cell count, so very little in the way of defense against anything, much less an aggressive adenovirus. She is coughing now. Each cough seems more wracking than the last.

An adenovirus invades a broad range of hosts and can cause life-threatening, multi-organ infection in people with weakened immune systems. They won't do the transplant if Linda has active, live virus in her system.

Rick retired from aerospace a few years ago. He teaches now as an adjunct professor at Antioch University in Los Angeles. He is an experimental cognitive psychologist who studies models of human behavior. A firm-featured, tall, and naturally fit man, he has a distinguished salt-and-pepper look softened by a professorial uniform of khakis and polo shirt. His computer roosts on a high drafting table in the den, at which we can find him during most waking hours, perched on his rolling stool, concentrating. From here, his agitation about Linda's cough is palpable. Our grief squeezes each of us privately.

It's my last night here. I'll go home tomorrow. Rick is harrying Linda about her cough. He can't help it, as if she were coughing on purpose, as if there is anything she can do. The virus rages on. Linda seems exasperated and defeated, both. The jig may be up. It's not her body's fault, but I think she is really very irritated, angry at her body. How could it betray her like this? I know Rick is frightened, too. He spends most of the day prodding his computer, preparing a review of a paper. Every time Linda sniffles or coughs, which she does more frequently each hour, he winces.

He has a class to teach tonight, so after dinner Linda and I have the evening to watch a show together. Truth be told, I'm frightened to be alone with all our feelings, but I also want to be available. My thoughts race and heat up, then shut down and shut up. The cycle repeats. We're just eating dinner, but all the fears, sadness, pain, and confusion about how to embrace this situation with some kind of equanimity fill my radio frequencies. It's hard for me to hear.

I try to start a conversation with Linda that will give her space and permission to voice any of her fears or feelings at the moment. I say something like, "It's not your fault that you have this cold." I've hit a sore spot. "Can we just watch a show and not talk? Please?" Linda says, lips tightening over a tight jaw.

Sunday. The cold has deepened overnight. The stem cells are waiting in a bag in a freezer, but Linda will not be able to think about using them until another six months from now. In the morning, I get ready to drive home. I feel like a giant hole has opened beneath us. I fear my sister will never be able to use those cells at all. When she walks me down the driveway to my car, we hug goodbye. We have not done that for a while; we've been respecting every immune-compromised cleanliness ritual in the book. We seem to have given up hope. I just want her to live, but today it seems impossible. She has a live tumor. She is barely alive herself after seven months of R-CHOP, but that fucking tumor is alive. And now she has a deadly adenovirus that knocked even stalwart Queen Elizabeth off her feet for weeks. She looks so forlorn. I'm sure I'll never see her again. We say goodbye with scratchy throats.

On the trip home, I howl. I don't know how I find the road beneath me. From the bottom of my heart, like a mama bear who has lost one of her babies to a prowling panther in a raging storm, I howl.

WHO AM I?

Santa Cruz Mountains
Spring 2017

I'm always the first one up at home, and I always go right downstairs for an eye-opening cup of black coffee. Fumbling with the K-Cup dispenser, I press the on switch. While waiting for the first shot to heat, I fill a carafe with filtered water from the spigot at the sink. I pour this into the water reservoir on the machine. The clear liquid slides in, silvery in the dull morning light. From an overhead cabinet, I take down a small cup and set it under the spout. I pop a pod of Peet's Major Dickason's Blend into the chamber. Pressing the down arrow to 6 OZ., I wait for the READY light and hit BREW.

Some say you should meditate before coffee so that your mind is calmer. I've given up trying to orchestrate my meditation experience. I am a terrible meditator, in that my mind never calms down and my moments of attending to silence are minuscule. The thing about grace is that is pierces the shield of your thoughts like a shard of sunlight startling through a parted curtain. Just a moment of resting in silence brings peace of mind that you don't forget. A partial second of inner silence can alter everything; it's enough. But first, I let the coffee cool until the smoky taste can fill my mouth without burning it.

I write an email to my cousin Joanne, the eldest of the kids in her family. "Don't ever do this to Holly and Ray," I say, referring to her younger brother and sister. I'm so mournful, I don't know what to say. "It's just hell." How would I ever get used to being alone here on earth without my big sister?

I take one mouthful. The taste of this coffee comes from hot-soaking roasted, ground-up berries gathered from plants growing halfway around the world. The harvest may have been years ago. Men and women, maybe children, plucked little red coffee beans from green plants on terraced hillsides, perhaps watered by little black hoses that run around each plant like decorative curlicues, or possibly by hand. Every one of these beans was collected, packaged, weighed, traded, shipped, and eventually roasted, ground, and packed into tiny plastic K-Cup pods. How many people and how many months and how many miles are involved in my cup of coffee? How many drops of rain fell on the little plant that supplied the beans that provide the roasted flavor rolling around in my mouth?

In 1985 I did a three-day retreat in the coastal woods of Northern California with Stephen Levine. Stephen was teaching from his book *Who Dies?* about the question "Who am I?" I wanted to connect with him and raised my hand with a question repeatedly, but he never called on me. Frustrated, I tracked him down on break. This was the early 1980s, when everyone was pretending they had quit smoking. So Stephen and I went out behind the main building and sat on the steps to the kitchen's rear entrance. We shook cigarettes out of our packs and lit up.

"I cry all the time. How do I release this grief and let it go?" I asked him.

"There is something in you that wants to be heard and felt," Stephen told me.

"I feel it all the time."

"No, it is consuming you; you are not hearing it. You are *being* it," he said.

I was stunned. I had never considered this before.

"You have to notice the feelings and embrace them as they arise, then let them pass. They must be known, or they will continue to overwhelm you."

"I see that," I said. "You're saying I could get enough space to embrace myself?"

"Yes. You have to mature into that. You have to be somebody before you can be nobody."

He was telling me not to destroy my individuality. It wanted to be experienced. The release we're seeking does not shut off or deny individuality; it embraces all of it. This was an invitation to heal by taking responsibility to move toward a more whole self-concept. Only I could do that for myself. "Come into yourself fully." Know thyself.

What am I, really?

I am the history of events that have occurred in my body. I am the ways I experience myself: sounds, visual images, colors, shapes, movement. I am the sensation of my body moving and knowing and smelling. I am the whole train of barely conscious thoughts that stream through my mind as I drive to the grocery store.

I am memories. I am a little kid who, on Sunday mornings, hoped this might be a Good Sunday, where my parents would read the paper together and Linda and I could lie on their bed and look at the color comics and dream of the day I could hold a newspaper and slap it into place like my dad. I am my high school prom, my college studies, the novels I've read.

I am my social roles: daughter, DOMPA, friend, mother, sister, employee, volunteer. I'm an organic, alive thing whose identity comes from interacting with other socially constructed identities. I was socially constructed in a family of wounded alcoholics, so I was originally rather poorly put together. I have core self-hatred that warped my early sense of self. But is there a way out? Can you find or generate within a more holistic, authentic sense of self? Yes, Buddha and I know there is a way. I can expand out of the depths somehow to include a more realistic sense of who I am.

On the floor in my den, I sit cross-legged on my little round *zafu*, black, with gold fire-breathing dragons. I take my right foot in my right hand and tuck it against my left calf under my thigh. Taking my left foot, I rest it on top of my right calf. If I keep my hips above my knees, I can sit still here for twenty or thirty minutes. I calm my mind with the meditative inquiry, "Who am I?" I let my attention go to the area behind my solar plexus. Then I want to find the sense of "I am." I try to remember what it feels like when I have a strong preference—I really love chocolate—and there is my sense of "I." I put attention on that and see what the sense of "I" is all about.

Sitting in silence, unmoving, I feel my being as a sense of vibrancy. I know I am alive. I am not *just* the passing thoughts. I am not *just* a fragmented self-concept. I am not merely this fear or that regret. I am not just my memories. I have this personality, and I have this unconscious mind, but what am I? I'm not really the witness, either, since I am aware of witnessing. I attend to the kinesthetic sensation in my belly, where I imagine a bulb of alive, silent being. Under the personality, there is a sense of brilliant, pulsing aliveness. What is *that*? I want to explore *that*.

The source of life is a real mystery. The source of my thoughts and emotions is a real mystery. They say that what you attend to, you will come to know. If I attend to these mysteries, will their vast silence penetrate me? After I listen to inner silence, my thoughts are more spacious and quiet. Thoughts come, thoughts go. "I am" remains. Feelings rise and dissipate. "I am" remains. I have found something stable within me. That is immeasurably reassuring.

In my senior years, I see that life is movement and change. You can't avoid troubles; being good does not protect you from disappointments, loss, or illness. I try to surf the waves these days, since I can't control them. Today, loss and grief are coming in waves that I can't control. I'm encountering the fact of change, the flowing nature of life. The mind stumbles weakly; my throat closes. It frightens me. I try to stay with the feeling and not the content of the thought. What is it really *like* to fear loss and death? Behind closed eyes, I feel desolation, falling through emptiness, nothing to grab onto. There is constriction in my throat and difficulty breathing. I feel . . . alone. It's the solitariness of it that strips me down; I feel like there is a howling wind whipping around me, but even in my imagination, I am just standing there in silence. The devastation is within. I allow that to roll through me and find it comes in waves. Eventually, it passes. I am alone. But I am not falling. I can flow with the flow, stay in my center of power in the middle of the heaves. I just have to keep finding my center, finding myself. Things quiet down and pass, and I wonder if I imagined the whole experience.

TRIAL

Los Angeles
April 2017

I f she has a serious viral infection, they're not going to give her the transplant. They have to take her immune system down to zero. If she has live virus in her, it will kill her. And she does have live virus. The transplant is canceled.

But by April 13, the virus is under control. Balancing risks versus possible outcomes, Dr. Zhou agrees to go ahead. We trust that he is committed to her survival, that she is likely to make it. So the transplant is back on.

It's just that her last chemo was a while ago, and that damn tumor is still alive.

One last check, a PET on Saturday, April 22, to check the activity of the tumor they have been blasting with the vile R-CHOP. The results, available on Monday, April 24, to Dr. Zhou, are bad. They show a live, hot, growing tumor. He will not proceed. The transplant is canceled.

What is going on? How did we get here? And now the options don't seem like real options. One: Linda tries another type of chemo, called RICE (rituximab, ifosfamide, carboplatin, etoposide), even more devastating than R-CHOP, and we see if she is alive at the end. Two: Linda gets a prescription for a mercy death, which helps her die in a few months. Three: She lands herself in one of the trials City of Hope is running. Linda has six days to decide and act. She gets moving.

Linda can't bear the thought of RICE. At some point, a person has to focus completely on herself to decide what she wants to do with the only life she has. We want Linda in our lives, but we have asked so much already. If she can't do RICE, that has to be okay with each of us. And "self-assisted death" is not an option Linda would actually choose at this point, so getting into a trial is the only way to go.

You'd think—and you'd be right—that the doctor at City of Hope would just assign Linda to an open trial and handle all the paperwork. But nothing is simple right now. Linda does get connected to a doctor running trials, and together they identify two or three that might work, but there are checklists; there are waitlists; there are protocols. She has to prove she meets the trial conditions, which are very specific regarding previous treatments and current health status. She's in a hurry; that tumor is growing and could outgrow the trial limits any minute. It's Tuesday, April 25. If she isn't in a trial by Monday, they're going to give her RICE next Tuesday.

Linda, having survived seven months of chemo and still at risk from that cold, crisscrosses the tangled freeways from Kaiser in LA to City of Hope in Duarte with records, files, films, results, approvals, lab reports, and memos, keeping everything moving from one desk to another. A deadline passes. An opening in a trial Linda wanted gets filled from a waitlist. Then a referral form seems to disappear. Linda makes distress calls to City of Hope administrators, and one finally responds to her insistence that the referral is somewhere in the system, if only they will find it. The helpful administrator tracks down the referral to the desk of the indifferent or inattentive Kaiser clerk who simply did not process the paperwork that could get Linda into that trial. Understanding the urgency, the City of Hope admin reboots the process. On Friday, April 28, we are down to one slot that closes Monday. Linda gets that slot. A victory—she's in a six-month trial! Jab effectively slipped.

On Thursday, May 4, Rick and Linda meet with Dr. Zain, the clinical-trial doctor at City of Hope. Everything is arranged. The trial protocol administers a targeted drug that eats B cell lymphoma tumors slowly but effectively. They will test her weekly for various kinds of tolerance and toxicity, which is what the trial is studying. They'll do this for six glorious, relatively easy, chemo-free months. At the end of that, she will have a tiny bit of tumor, maybe dead or maybe alive. But if there is no live virus, she will get the transplant.

My checklist is growing.

- Viable donor

- Perfect match

- Get into trial to stay alive until transplant

- Complete trial

- Get transplant

- Transplant succeeds

- No graft versus host (GVH) disease!

- Heal completely

- Kill tumor

TRIAL VISIT

Los Angeles
August 2017

The trial protocol is effective. The tumor shrinks within days; Linda can feel it. The drug—called an antibody-drug conjugate (ADC)—delivers a cytotoxic poison that kills cells, just like the chemotherapy, but it has a lifesaving feature. The antibody part can find cells with a special marker—the C-22 marker. Markers are sticky proteins on the outside of a cell membrane. The HLA markers that match in us 10/10 are the same type of thing—sticky marker proteins. The C-22 marker is on B cells. The trial drug finds cells with the C-22 marker. Instead of carpet-bombing your system and killing all fast-growing cells, such as those in your intestinal lining or hair follicles, this drug delivers the payload to B cells. That has the unwelcome side effect of wiping out your active immune response, but it's a lot easier to tolerate than general-purpose chemotherapy.

There is other collateral damage. Linda's body will bear the impact in partial loss of lung capacity and damage to her kidneys, liver, and maybe eyes. But she is recovering from chemo. The tumor is shrinking. She is alive and moving in the right direction. She is able to do things she could not do during regular chemo. She is not continually nauseated and does not succumb to opportunistic infections.

One week during this six months of trial therapy, I drive into town for a visit. I expect to find, upon entering Linda and Rick's home, that life hangs perilously and we whisper. But things are completely different from the last time I was here. The atmosphere is upbeat and far less burdened. Linda has energy and Rick is at ease. We go swimming in the blue oval backyard pool. They're using a Port-a-Cath buried under Linda's skin to administer the trial drug, so she can submerge herself in the soothing, cooling water. We spin in circles, do laps in easy breaststroke, and drift. There is a family of chatty parrots who have taken residence in the tall coconut palms that tremble over Linda's yard. They have some friends over for the afternoon. They are green with a bright orange or red splash on the head, and they make bright, happy chirps. We snoop on them from under our hats, Linda's a Lucky Brand floppy straw, mine a blue cap with the lettering THINK OUTSIDE.

We can feel the pressure of the water against our muscles as we spin, twisting our legs in big circles under us. Our arms move in big loops or back and forth, back and forth. We float on our backs on foam noodles from Alaia's big can full of pool toys.

Ari visits Linda and Rick on Saturdays. Today he drove over with his laundry, after playing hockey in the morning. Some days he finds his mom napping, some days playing chess, some days reading. Previous days she had rich, long, brushed-back hair or she was bald. Today she is in a stubble phase, several months into the trial. He always greets her with an energetic smile, a big, warm hug, and ready laughter. Ari is a vigorous guy. He probably swam in the Santa Monica Bay this morning after dawn, maybe dashing among a pod of dolphins. He exudes confidence in Linda's strength; I think he has never doubted she will kick this thing.

Ari played basketball, tennis, and Ultimate Frisbee until an injury forced a change. Now it's swimming and ice hockey. Muay Thai is my first sport, really, so I appreciate that Ari, a general-purpose athlete, can talk boxing with me a little. I have high hopes for Conor McGregor in the upcoming McGregor-Mayweather boxing match in Vegas. I show Ari some of the moves I think Conor, coming from mixed martial arts and kickboxing, could make on Floyd, a pure boxer. Ari keeps an open mind, but he probably knows there's a slim chance Mayweather will lose. It's a pure boxing match, and Floyd Mayweather has forty-nine wins and zero losses in his career. None of us is a boxing aficionado, but the energy of sports is entertaining and we are all interested. I show Linda and Rick a YouTube demonstration of ways in which Conor could land devastating punches on Floyd.

Rick tells me he explained to his students about his wife's struggle with lymphoma. Of course they responded with genuine concern, and I think this is comforting for Rick. You have to talk with other people about your pain, or it gets worse. You have to let people in and recall you are not alone. When you realize everyone has something to face, it softens you.

Rick invites a couple over for dinner, a research fellow he knew from RAND Corporation and his wife, a medical doctor. He grills some flank steak outside by the pool. The meat has been marinating for several hours in the kitchen, and now that it is cooking, charring at the edges, even my vegetarian mouth is watering. Flank steak on toasted hard rolls with A.1. Sauce is an old family favorite, with thin-sliced purple onion. One of Mom's specialties. I haven't had it in many years, since my daughter converted me to a lower-stress diet. I grill a piece of vegetarian chik'n made with mycoprotein and whey. It makes a great sandwich.

Linda makes an appetizer and a side dish, I've forgotten what. The point is, she is up cooking and is having company. This is life; this is what she wanted to do, instead of be dead. We are on a roll.

We eat outside under the canopy after we all get in the pool and goof around. Linda is relaxed and laughing. We all are. None of us drinks; nothing is going to happen later. There will be no arguments, no violence, no hatred. We enjoy food and company. We laugh and tell stories and explain our ideas to each other. I stay pretty centered in my Zenny Zone. Life couldn't be better.

Linda tells me later, with genuine surprise, that she really enjoyed dinner and my presence. She hadn't been able to socialize during chemo. She appreciated that I was good company. That's charming to hear, except the implication stings. It's just sad to learn that all these years, I thought we were such good friends, while Linda kind of expected not to enjoy my company. I have to keep resetting my world to get my thoughts to line up with reality. I've been living in fantasy worlds. Now I am getting the chance to realign. You suffer, they say, only so far as you struggle with what's so.

TRANSPLANT

DAY ZERO: FULL CIRCLE

City of Hope
Duarte
October 2017

Linda lazily expected that the six-month trial would extend into a one-year trial. But no, it ends in October, and Linda is really in much better shape than she was six months ago after chemo. All the conditions are set for transplant, so it's time to do it.

They perform a surgery to install a Hickman line, a tube going into a large vein in the chest, just above the heart. To any normal person, the installation of the port would be a major bodily intrusion and violation. To a patient with the patience it takes to be a successful patient, it's just another step in a long walk. The pre-transplant chemo, the transplant chemo, the transplant, blood stabilizers, and everything else is going down that tube into that vein. And you would be correct in thinking that there is a type of designer chemo for every need.

Pre-transplant chemo starts eleven days prior as an outpatient treatment. Linda goes into City of Hope for the infusion. Eight days prior to the transplant, on Monday, October 16, Linda goes into a sterile isolation room at City of Hope. She will be in here for a month.

Lise Mathews, of Linda's Divine Book Club, which earns its nickname through the inspired buttressing they give Linda and Rick, posters the walls of Linda's room with photos of her loved ones. She has a small window looking out on the campus, through which she can observe the changing of day and night. Beneath this porthole is a green faux-leather club chair that visitors will use.

My nephew, Ari, has read testimonials of transplant survivors to discover what small amenities might ease various discomforts, and he makes Linda a survivor pack that joins her knitting, Kindle, and audiobooks in the bedside table drawers. Her bed faces a television that will never be turned on, and a whiteboard where her daily stats will be tallied. A bedside potty is tucked against the bed for easy access. Pressed by the whiteboard stands a nurses' table packed with Linda's chart, a box of latex gloves, and bleachy Handi Wipes. When the curtain around her bed is pulled back, Linda can look through a hallway window out onto a folding table with a chair where visitors can eat lunch. Linda purchases meal tickets ahead of time for her guests. We can then order lunch from a California-fresh menu of healthy foods. But we can't eat in the room with Linda because of the isolation protocols. Visitors wear masks in the isolation rooms.

Finally, we are at the critical moment. Boom shakalaka. The boom: Pre-transplant nuclear-bomb chemo—fludarabine with melphalan as a reduced-intensity myeloblastic conditioning regime for an allo-geneic hematopoietic stem cell transplant. It is designed to maintain the graft-versus-malignancy effect. This shit kills bone marrow. The shakalaka: the stem cell infusion on Day Zero, Tuesday, October 24. Cope medical staff call this Linda's new birthday.

A miracle of Western medicine unfolds over the next one hundred days: keeping Linda alive, without bone marrow or immunity or red blood cells, while letting the transplant take root and grow.

This is magical alchemy of which Dr. Farol, now her transplant doctor instead of Zhou, is a skilled practitioner. Although it is called a "reduced-intensity" regimen, Linda loses her hair and her appetite and her energy for nearly three months. She does not, however, lose her sense of humor, her will to live, or her love of opera.

Lise Mathews sets up a visitation schedule with the Divine Book Club, so Linda has guests every day. Some days she does not want to see people, but later, when she is able to get up and start her walks, she will remember that these visits kept her going and pulled her through. The medical team tells her that "many visitors" correlates highly with rapid recovery.

There are days of progress and setbacks. No serious issues arise. Everything is working; it's just a painful and slow process. The new system is settling in; it is making new blood cells, red and white. We won't know for a few weeks if this stuff is from the transplant, but all looks good. She's getting immunosuppressants to prevent this new immune system from mustering an attack on her host cells—that would mean the graft is attacking the host. It's a balancing act.

She has difficulty eating food and keeping it down. She seems like she would be pretty miserable moment by moment, but she gets through it all quietly. I don't know what goes through her mind. Perhaps the drug cocktail has mercifully supplied some antianxiety medication to help her cruise. Her white blood cell count is rising steadily—WBC: 0.5, 0.7, 1.1.

I keep waiting for the Big Setback. Everything I read suggests there are so many risks that the chances of her getting out of here alive are crummy. Organ failures, infections, rejection. There are far more ways this can go wrong than right. But Linda has already made it past most of the problems that I find on the Internet. Are we going to really make it? Can we exhale?

For a few days, there is concern that Linda is harboring C. difficile bacteria, which they can treat with antibiotics but which also pose a risk to others. While this is a concern, we have to cover up with masks, caps, and gowns while inside her room; on the way out, we strip them off and discard them in the biohazard bin at the door. On normal days, we need to wear masks in the room to protect Linda, but not the capes and caps, which were to isolate the C. difficile. Nursing staff are able to manage so many things using various straightforward protocols like this. There is no rushing about dealing with surprises. They really have this down.

There is a period when Linda swells up from an imbalance in her blood chemistry. It takes the medical team a few days to get the right balance of electrolytes so she can start releasing fluid that's gotten trapped in her body tissues. She can't eat at all, but eventually this works itself out. Soon, she is on schedule with all the recovery steps:

- Walking daily

- Eating daily

- WBC count rising

- Stable blood chemistry

If she keeps this up, she'll be home by Day Thirty for sure. Happy birthday, dear Linda. Happy birthday to you.

VISITING THE COPE

City of Hope
Duarte
Fall 2017

Day Ten. I drive down to LA to spend a week visiting Linda at City of Hope. The night before I go in, Rick and I order a pizza and watch the Dodgers play in the World Series. We drink a couple of St. Pauli Girl nonalcoholic beers, like a couple of ordinary people without a crisis/miracle going on.

The next morning, I stay to the left on the motorways and get to City of Hope around 9:00 a.m. I find a parking spot and walk over to the transplant building, take the elevator up, and follow the signs. After touching anything, I squirt some hand sanitizer from an automatic dispenser into my palm and brush it over my hands. When I arrive, I peek at Linda through the lunchtime window. She looks so innocent and vulnerable, sleeping there in her transplant bed, that I can see the child inside the woman. She's been poisoned and lived to tell about it. Her face, previously swollen like a pumpkin, today looks more like a grape. The excess water is dissipating. They have given her a full blood transfusion to raise her hemoglobin levels and adjusted the immunosuppressants downward.

I gown up before going in. We have some kind of extra contain-
ment protocol going on today. I put on a gown, a mask, and latex
gloves. I choose size S for my small hands, but I rip the thin, stretchy
film as I pull it over my knuckles. I switch to size M. I've come to
sit with her a few days. I'm not sure she really wants the company.
I'm hard to get rid of, though, and she said I could come. She looks
like what she's going through. I hope my presence will cheer her, but
inside I feel kind of frozen. I hope I can relax and stop worrying
about her while I'm here. I hope she feels uplifted, at least befriended.
You don't always feel befriended in a family; sometimes it's all old
patterns and defenses. In our family, you had to be on your defensive
toes.

My parents made fun of us for no reason, or for entertainment.
Dad liked to insult women, just to enjoy his own wit. And you were
supposed to enjoy it with him, enjoy seeing him enjoying himself
insulting you, or Mom, or Linda. In a sense, it was his profession, as a
comedy writer in touch with the times. Later on, I would understand
some of his humor in a cultural context, as backlash by white men
against the empowerment and employment women achieved during
the war years. But the child took what Daddy said as facts about the
nature of girls and women.

My father was a natural in the misogynist-humor movement.
Derisive put-downs were just the thing for the narcissist in him. I
had heard him abuse women, including my mother, with drunken,
foul-mouthed invectives. I can still feel the way he teased Linda when
she was only ten or eleven. She was dressing to go to a children's
opera with Mother. *Is he making fun of her and it's supposed to be
funny? Why doesn't Mother do something?* By the time Linda was
thirteen, she couldn't take it anymore and went away to a Catholic
girls' boarding school. Can you imagine that being an improvement?

—

Medical staff move in and out of the room continually. The IV machine starts to beep, too loudly. "Oh, it beeps almost every fifteen minutes," Linda says. "I'm just learning how to sleep so it won't go off. It's very sensitive."

Alicia presses a button and fiddles with one tube. "A line tends to get clogged," she apologizes. Juan, Alicia, Ellen, and Robert all cheerfully come and go, checking and updating. There are some additives to Linda's blood today: diuretics, electrolytes. They put the stuff right into her Hickman port. In these early weeks, we are waiting for the stem cells to implant. The first few days, they drifted in Linda's bloodstream until they resettled in her bone marrow, where, we hope, they found nourishment, settled down, and started multiplying. That takes about ten days. The healthier the cells, the better the implant.

These cells make the precursors for red and white blood cells. I had done my best to make them potent, vigorous, and productive. She will have my blood type, O negative. Since that is the universal-donor blood type, it will cause no problems in her previously A-positive system. The WBCs become the components of the new immune system. We watch the numbers start to go up on the whiteboard every morning. WBC: 1.7, 2.3, 2.7. It looks like the implant has rooted. Could she be on the mend? You go one day at a time with transplants.

One of the days, I read aloud from a classic horror story, *The Haunting of Hill House*, by Shirley Jackson. After all, it is the Halloween season. Linda loves to read out loud. She taught me how to read by reading to me. My favorite and the most fascinating book in our home was *The Magical Land of Noom*, about a couple of kids who, through their own imaginative powers, make a magical journey to the dark side of the moon. Linda read all of those words to me, and by the end, I could read them myself. For her fiftieth birthday, I scrounged around among antique booksellers and found an ancient copy of it. I was nearly forty-eight years old before I realized that *Noom* is *Moon* spelled backward.

We all like to read, but Daddy joked that he liked to read so much, he'd read the advertising on cereal boxes. He had an entire wall made into shelves for books in the den. It was my favorite place in the house.

Summer 1960

Mysteries of life and science and history and ideas that drive everything out in the big world must have been hidden in the rising rows of books that marched in the space above my nine-year-old head. I hoped to devour them all someday. But then I was learning to read the kids' books. I loved the Hardy brothers, Joe and Frank. I struggled through their adventures with devotion. I could watch them on *The Mickey Mouse Club*, too. My father collected all the volumes in the series, which he read as a child. I also loved the tales of sci-fi wonder Tom Swift Jr., son of the marvelous Tom Swift of my father's childhood. But today I took down *The Big Book of Fun*.

Linda was usually the one who did the construction projects in this book, but that afternoon I taught myself how to make a magic wand using a hanger dowel, construction paper, scissors, and glue. The trick was to make two wands. One was black construction paper wrapped around a cardboard hanger dowel, with white paper around the tip. The second, a trick wand only, had only a short dowel in the magical tip at the end, so I could tap it on the table and it would sound solid. Really, the trick wand was just rolled-up black construction paper. I learned how to make the trick wand disappear in newspaper, then reappear in my sleeve, and I practiced the magic trick so I could show Daddy the next time he came home. Sometimes he went missing for a couple of days. I showed Mommy, and because she couldn't do magic like Daddy could, she was totally fooled. I couldn't wait to show him.

The main thing with magic tricks was to tell a story the whole time that would distract your audience from the real thing going on.

The story was called the "patter." You could say you were traveling in this strange, foreign land when you came upon this magical wand, or mirror, or deck of cards. I came across my disappearing wand while wandering among the camels in the hot sands of Egypt.

Meantime, Linda was training me to be a prince. I must have announced once to her that I wanted to be king of the world and fix everything. Linda convinced me that before I could be king I had to be a prince, and princes had to learn a lot of stuff—English and history and math and things Linda knew.

Linda prepared study sheets of things I had to learn. Names of countries and their capitals. Works of famous people like Shakespeare. Addition with carrying. She wrote out the lessons by hand. At the end of my study period, she gave me a test. Ardent in my desire to be a good king, I did well on each day's exam.

After a while, we had to decide whether to play clubhouse with our stuffed animals, read books, or do other stuff. I wanted to play outside, so I got my Winchester cap rifle and ran into my front yard to join a band of cowboys who were chasing bad guys through the wild canyons there. I ran out of ammunition, so I had to fashion a bow and arrow from the sticks I found in the yard. Under a willow tree, I broke off a good, strong stick that I could bend into a bow. I used a simple string for my catgut bowline. I stole a knife from the kitchen to whittle my little arrows to points. I left out feathers, as I had no idea how I would add those. Anyway, the string didn't really launch the arrows. But I was able to defend myself until I got back to the saloon.

On Sunday morning, I watched TV quietly in the den beneath the built-in bookshelves, hoping my parents would sleep in and we could skip Mass. You had to adjust the rabbit-ears antennae to get the best picture. I loved Timmy on *Lassie*, and *The Little Rascals*, *Adventures of Superman*, and *The Swamp Fox*. I wished Linda would come in and watch with me.

—

Although I would have somehow learned to read without Linda, I still owe her. Today, by reading her Jackson's spooky novel, I can pay that forward just a little.

Elizabeth and I plan to have dinner together for her sixtieth birthday, which will be coming up in a couple of days. She and her best buddy Dana will go out of town, running up the coast on the 101 to Santa Barbara for a girlfriends' weekend of museums, beaches, shops, and restaurant-bars. Dana's been a family friend since Beth was in grade school; she's been there through our thicks and our thins. She and my sister will make each other laugh and stay light-hearted. On Tuesday, after I visit Linda at City of Hope, I book it out of there to brave the LA freeway system and chug on out toward Culver City to meet Beth.

LA is a city of evolving neighborhoods. Culver City is on the rise, fresh places to eat emerging as the town attracts the new Californians spilling out of Silicon Beach and Venice to the west. We're meeting at the Venice–Culver City border for Thai food. I take the 605 route, hoping to bypass the worst congestion on the 101. But I end up driving by the new Dodger Stadium. I forgot: Tonight is the stadium's first World Series—Game Seven of Dodgers versus Astros. Dodgers will lose it 5–1 during dinner. For which I am late.

But it's a treat for us to have time alone, away from other family dynamics, with good food and things to celebrate: Beth's birthday, Linda's recovery, my happiness with the transplant result so far. We meet at Natalee Thai on Venice Boulevard. Beth already has Thai wraps on the table waiting for me and rises to hug me with a warm smile. She wants to hear about the drive and my time with Linda and anything I want to talk about. Her hair curls in a cute new cut around her little, animated face. We take a few minutes to look at the menu, and then we decide on spicy eggplant and *maha jumlong* curry. Bethy laughs as she teases me about being a hero. Must be exhausting, taking all that thanks and praise, she pokes. But, more seriously, she asks if I will feel lost without this purpose in my life.

"How's that going to be, no big purpose driving you?"

I scoff. Pshaw—who needs purpose? Then I wonder about it for the rest of dinner. "You're probably right, Bethy. I'm going to feel kind of lost. I wonder what I'll do. I hope I don't decide to take actual fights."

"They let people your age fight?"

"Yeah, they don't have a big structure around this sport. You sign consent forms. My doctors say I'm healthy. So it's up to me."

What are my intentions now? I do better when I have clear intentions. What would I get out of a fight, other than proving I was brave enough—or stupid enough—to do it? My brother-in-law Len, who loves boxing but does not box himself, says, "You should do it! What could happen, really? How bad could it be?"

It's only two two-minute rounds. But is kickboxing with a live opponent a real aspiration of mine? I don't think I actually want to hurt someone. That could be a problem for me as a fighter.

We pile on the appetizers and the main course and get more than we can put away, and it's delightful. We take note of the depressing score of the final game in the World Series, which I can see on the TV across the room, over Bethy's shoulder. There's nothing to fix, no one to save, nobody dying. It seems like Beth and I haven't had a night off like this in twenty years.

It was less than a year and a half ago on June 27 that Mom died. Bethy was caretaking at Mom's house. She was determined to help Mom have a shower. She wrapped her arms around Mom gently, under the arms, putting Mom's hands around her neck. This way, Bethy could help her into the stall, where handles and a bench provided stabilizers. Mom had become resistant about the shower, maybe because of her tender, neuropathic skin, but she usually gave up resistance eventually. As Bethy lifted, Mom's body gave out a big sigh and collapsed into Beth. They both landed on the floor. She had slipped away a bit more.

Bethy got her back to bed, tucked in with warm blankets, and tried to keep her hydrated. Mom would sip through a straw. Bethy massaged Mom's slight muscles through the blanket. Then she went into the kitchen, perhaps to prepare a snack or some tea. It was the late afternoon. Privately, quietly, Mommy died. No death throes. When Elizabeth came back into the room, she found a completed, silent, gone Mommy. They stayed there together awhile before calling us.

Elizabeth has been able to get back into her own life successfully. Whatever she completed with Mom is serving her now. I can feel the confidence and centeredness growing in her. Bethy has been to the hinterland and back, and she really does not need anyone's bullshit anymore, thank you. We share some war stories about our daily lives, confessing our discomfort with anger or celebrating the ability to let go of a misplaced feeling of responsibility. We are practicing boundaries, the both of us. We share some tactics we use to deal with people who treat us with disrespect. You can't force people to respect you, but you can disconnect from reacting to their bullshit. Beth tells some pretty funny stories about ways to ignore someone's ravings while focusing on the tasks at hand. I feel like I am seeing her for the first time, after she has emerged as a wise woman into her own life. A real force to be reckoned with.

Happy birthday, dear Elizabeth. Happy birthday to you.

The City of Hope annual fundraising walk is this week. They will raise over $1 million on Sunday, November 5. Elizabeth plans to do the walk. She sets her fundraising goal, but within a couple of days she has doubled it, then tripled it. By the time she finishes, she has raised ten times her goal. That Sunday afternoon, she stops by the isolation room for a visit after the walk.

"I can't believe you just did that, right while I'm in here." Linda beams at Bethy. She is moved, again, to tears. They flow more freely nowadays.

"It was a fun walk," Beth says. "Very upbeat, people all here for a good reason."

"Thank you so much, Elizabeth," Linda says, stricken for a moment with the immensity of what is going on.

Linda's machine beeps again. Sometimes we let it beep, or Linda buzzes a nurse to come reset it. They do this repeatedly without cursing or kicking the damn thing. Alicia comes in to clear the line. You can't stay mad at it; the apparatus is like a lifesaving soda machine. It mixes and delivers an ever-changing cocktail of healing agents that keep Linda alive. A man whose sole responsibility is machine health comes in multiple times daily to verify the correct working of its electronics.

At this stage, an unsuppressed, rebooted immune system would try to mount a campaign against Linda's body cells. Likely targets would be intestinal lining, eyes, mouth, and skin. We see no signs of this, but if it got started and ran out of control, it would be deadly serious. Many chemicals that you and I pay no attention to have to be balanced and kept within certain parameters to ward off dangerous conditions. Alicia marks notes in the chart on the stand by the whiteboard, checks the numbers, cheerfully asks Linda a few questions. The caustic trace of chlorine from the bleach wipes bites into the air. The whiteboard still shows yesterday's numbers.

Another day, Linda suggests we listen to highlights from opera. Her kids will later call this a true act of devotion, but it's actually very moving. Plus, Linda is merciful and selects pieces that could crack a stone's heart. You want to bring a light attitude to the whole situation—like this nursing staff does!—but this is heavy stuff. Opera takes you on a passage through the extremes of sentiment, so what better way to engage with what is really happening—extremes.

Each time Linda selects an aria, she tells me the story in general and then describes the particular scene at hand. I close my eyes and let myself be carried on the sound waves. She plays arias on her phone, connected to a mini Bluetooth speaker she brought just for this. "*O mio babbino caro*"; "*Nessun dorma*," ending with several moving repetitions of *Vincerò!* ("I will prevail!"); and "*Voi che sapete*." We go through all her favorites. Just sitting there in a hospital, surrounded by white and machines, you can be stretched out into deep yearning, shattered by love, dropped into the depths of loss, or sent alone into the abyss to meet the truth. The afternoon nurse, Alicia, remarks how beautiful one aria is. It makes us weep. How much better for the soul than daytime TV. We go on like this for hours and hours.

Everyone at City of Hope is relating to terminal illness one way or another. We are all in the same boat. In the outside world, we can forget we will all eventually die. Here, many patients wear headscarves; some wear masks. No one is coughing or sneezing, and the rare exception seems loud and intrusive. Visitors rarely have colds; they ask you not to come if you have any symptoms. People move slowly and are friendly, often smiling. When we make eye contact, they are present. Rising from the depths of absorption with our own struggles, we are kind to each other. We move through an atmosphere different from that of the outside world. We are not competing with each other in a zero-sum game. At work, everyone seems to aspire to outdo the next person. Here, we are all in similar rough spots.

City of Hope has great survival statistics, and you get the impression people like their jobs and that their patients tend to live. If you come into the main building, you pass the Spirit of Life fountain. The sculpture's exuberant parents toss their child in handheld happy play drenched in what looks like the sound of laughter. They make a vibrant circle, inviting you to raise your spirits to the Spirit of Life standard. Spots of serenity and beauty, including an open, well-lit library, make it possible to walk around the cancer center without getting blue. Actually, people here are on positive trajectories; most of them are getting better. You have the feeling that you are in a healthier, more positive, and intentional environment at City of Hope than at, for example, Walmart.

DINNER PARTY

Santa Cruz Mountains
November 2017

After a weeklong visit, I drive home early one morning. As the Toyota weathers the 405 out of LA, a rare rainstorm is brewing and we both keep going until I merge with Interstate 5 North in a downpour. Raindrops bang loudly on my windshield, and I stay in the second-to-right lane, taking my time, along with the trucks grinding down their gears to pull themselves up the mountain. I have nowhere else to be. Thick sprays from passing traffic's rear tires drench my windshield. Dense layers of dark rainclouds like Brillo pads rise up to the north and east. I-5 takes you up the Grapevine toward Wheeler Ridge. Up there, you pass on your left, to the west, the peaks surrounding Mt. Pinos in the Los Padres National Forest. Those are the peaks where my mom and Hank lived, and, I kid you not, they are ablaze with orange and gold as I drive past them in this dark, battering storm. First of all, how often does the high desert outside LA get a storm? Climate change brings them about now and then, but this one is a doozy. But I swear, to the northwest over the Mt. Pinos cluster where Mom and Hank died last year, as I drive up one of the sweeping curves into the view, I see the sky ripped open by great gashes of brilliant light—yellow gold and white, slashed with pink and bright orange, flaming—and framed by masses of billowy white clouds. Mommy is really proud of us. Her heart is bursting with light to let us know she is with us. I knew she would be.

This year, I want to throw a dinner party for Jill. She is turning fifty-five, and I have pretty much ignored her for the past year and a half. I think I'll do a big sheet of vegetarian lasagna or eggplant Parmesan, with a tossed salad and garlic bread. Sitting in Ari's old bedroom in Linda's house, I had gotten things started. I sent the invitations out secretly so that Jill would not find out prematurely. I want to try bringing together friends and family who don't normally mix. Jill's family and their families are one group, my daughter and Jill's trans godson and their partners are another, our gay friends make a third, and several neighbors comprise a fourth. Mixing these people is going to be great.

I wait until I know at least twelve people are coming; we'll have a real sit-down dinner at the dining room table that looks as festive as a holiday. I've never hosted a dinner party for this many people, though. I know I'm not going to be able to pull off a surprise. So I mention it casually one morning over coffee in bed.

"Oh, Jill, we're having a dinner party for your birthday on November twelfth. I thought I'd do pasta."

She glances up from her iPad in surprise. "Why?"

"For your birthday." *What an odd response*, I think.

"Why for my birthday?" She seems embarrassed, or shy!

"A party for you. Just because." Because life is so vulnerable; because you could go out like that. *Snap!*

"My family?"

"Yes, all of them, and Tristan and Christie, and Lucy, Karen,

Illana, Jan. Mark. Your niece and nephew." I am happy everyone is coming so I can see the smile take over her face. "We should probably get something from Gail's," she says, and I know we are good to go.

We do the lasagna and the eggplant. We order the lasagna from Gail's and start the eggplant the night before. Jill helps me cook; well, really, I help her. We stay up late, slicing the eggplant into rounds and salting it on paper towels. Jill dips each piece in beaten egg and bread crumbs before we bake the rounds in the oven at 375 degrees. We listen to the Grateful Dead and sing "Ripple" and "Casey Jones" off-key, which makes us right in tune with Jerry. Crispy slices stack up, golden brown, plump, and juicy. Tomorrow, we will layer these into a baking dish with handfuls of shredded mozzarella and Parmesan cheese and drench it all in marinara sauce.

Sunday evening, our guests arrive, bearing wine and gifts. Most of the folks have met once or twice or have heard of each other. I, of course, don't drink, and the guests are moderate, appropriate drinkers who will have, at most, two glasses of wine. This is enough to slightly lower the social stressors. People are comfortable and chatty. The mix works out really well, stimulating lots of conversation about what is going on in everyone's life.

"How is Linda doing?" our brother-in-law Lenny asks, and Jill, beaming and proud of us, answers, "It's amazing, Len. She's doing really well." Suddenly, she is crying. "It's all about family," she is saying, "and showing up for them and loving your family and friends." She raises a toast to family and friends, and we all get a little weepy. "To life!" we cry out.

I am secretly thinking of a little joke I have with Linda. If she were here, I would say, "To wives and sweethearts—may they never meet." And we would both know the book series this comes from, about the adventures of Jack Aubrey and Stephen Maturin, by Patrick O'Brian. Or I might sing a line from a childhood Broadway musical or recall an image from *Winnie-the-Pooh*. Perhaps I'm obnoxious, but I love these little jokes we've been making since I could talk, our little connections. And I love Linda so.

Most of the time when Jill's family comes over, they do the dishes and clean up after we eat. But tonight they are guests at our dinner party and I don't let them help. I clear plates, and we make room for dessert. I've got a creamy red-velvet layer cake from Santa Cruz's finest bakery, the Buttery. When I bring out the cake we of course sing, "Happy birthday, dear Jill, happy birthday to you."

Eventually I move everyone into the family room, where Jill has to open her presents like a little kid, with everyone watching. She is self-conscious but also elated—she's been laughing and talking and singing all night. After most people go home, a few close and local friends stay. We talk, animated and gesturing, into the night. I forget for a few minutes about life and death.

DAY TWENTY-THREE

Los Angeles
November 2017

On Day Twenty-Three, Linda comes home!

The day is foggy in my memory. I remember that I borrow Jill's Porsche and chug out of the chilly Santa Cruz Mountains as the first orange-pink light breaks across the Loma Prieta ridge. The little roadster hums through the light traffic; the only people on the roads at that hour are nurses and road construction workers. Driving this vacation car with the buttery leather interior makes cruising feel like a visit to the spa. Maneuvering along Interstate 5 through the Grapevine is easy like creamy vanilla-bean ice cream, and I get to the 405 and into West LA before the afternoon commuter gridlock. I go to the Whole Foods on National. I asked Rick how I could help, and he suggested I get dinner for the two of us and a few items that Linda might eat. He and Linda will be checking out of City of Hope early this afternoon.

I pick something Linda can eat, but there's so little. A mouthful of yogurt? Applesauce? Perhaps a potato. I don't recall. I also get something I can easily put together for Rick and me, maybe a frozen lasagna. I stow my grocery bags in the backseat and slide into the driver's pocket. The key snickers into the ignition—on the left of the steering column in this German car—but will not turn when I torque it, so I can't get the car to start, and there's a construction crew next to the parking lot, cutting vast sheets of metal with an impossibly loud screeching blade that cuts the air into wild, screaming strips, and I start to panic. Then I remember I cannot give in to that. So I get my breath steady and my legs under me and regain my composure. I call home to Jill; she's the strength and stability in my life and knows what to do in crises. Plus, this is her car. What the fuck is wrong with it?

She doesn't know. Call AAA, she says. Fifteen years ago, it would have been AA, but all right. My heart is hammering along with the screeching metal, and I'm sweating, but, dammit, I will call. But won't the food start to go bad and Linda can't have any germs festering in any food it all has to be so fresh and clean and now the food is in my car in LA heat even though it is November so not that bad but wait maybe the Divine Book Club can help. I call Lise Mathews, and I think my voice is skipping beats. Can she help get these groceries to Linda and Rick's house? I am riding waves of queasiness, breathing as it goes through me, knowing I cannot lose control and mess this up, knowing eventually my mind will slow down and I will figure out what to do. I can buy new groceries. It would work. I count in my head while Lise explains to me about LA traffic and the impossibility and it is a workday and relatives for the Thanksgiving holiday and . . . I am embarrassed, but I remember maybe I should not feel ashamed to ask for help, but then shame floods me anyway. I apologize and hang up as fast as I can. I promise to call next time I need something.

Yet the gods of transplants smile on me. Unzipping the side pocket of my purse, I fumble out my wallet and am sliding out my AAA card when Jill calls back. "Okay, it's a steering-wheel lock mechanism; a security thing. If you pull on the wheel after you park, it locks it in place. Harder to steal." She explains how to jerk the wheel to unjam it. My breath is in tatters, sweat douses me, but, dang it, I am getting these groceries home on time. I did not mess this up. I back out of that tiny LA parking spot and squish onto National, easily attaining Westwood and finding my way onto Santa Monica Boulevard. Things flow smoothly in my direction. In LA, if you plan it out, you can move nicely from neighborhood to neighborhood. Fortunately, this straight ride down Santa Monica does not require my attention in any way; I know the route to Linda's house.

Linda's house is a place where I have tried to claim ground. When I was little, I lacked a basic sense of stability. I was always trying to find a place where I belonged—someplace or somebody I could grab onto, like banisters on my life stairs. Not until middle age would I understand that stability comes from within, from a stable, consistent, and fairly whole concept of self. But in my thirties and forties, I could never seem to get any permanent banisters. That very desperation would make me feel even more hopeless. A couple of times a year, I'd go visit Linda to get restabilized. It was only years later, now, that I understood she might have felt a little invaded. I needed to get my own stabilizers, which didn't really happen until I came out of that millennium depression, in my sixties.

In AA they used to say we alkies had a god-size hole inside. God knows it felt like it. It was an ache of loneliness, or isolation, or futility—as if the whole story of your life just kept collapsing and throwing you out the window. You were just always falling. As I matured, I would see this loss of ground as a kind of opening or opportunity to befriend myself, even this empty confusion in me. But, since Linda was our generation's matriarch, the firstborn of all the cousins, I (inappropriately, I think now) tried to make her home into a safe center for myself. But today I understand I am a visitor here. I have to bring my own banisters.

I am familiar with the feeling of not finding any ground to stand in, of the rug being pulled out, and of falling. I comfort myself with the memory that I've faced falling before and know how to fall gracefully. I can trust myself to get up. I always get through. Worst case, you just put your chin down and stay tight. You can get through anything. But I pray I can offer more than just getting through it in the days to come. *Please help me be a good sister and companion and support them without being annoying.*

I pull into their driveway to unload the car, then move my car out to the street. I'll have to remember to get a parking pass from Rick. Each neighborhood has restricted parking. He will pull the Prius into the driveway to the sidewalk nearest the door so Linda won't have to walk far. But she's been walking the isolation ward quite a bit. At City of Hope, the transplant patients have to get up with all their IVs and whatnot to walk around the unit as soon as they can. After you walk the full cycle to the exit and back, you get to collect a little rubber foot to add to your chain. You have to collect as many little rubber feet as you possibly can. Linda pushed herself like the dogged Hungarians she descended from. She had lots of little feet. But when they arrive and Rick pulls the car up and she gets out to walk to the house, she stumbles on the driveway blacktop.

"Goddammit," Rick curses. It's probably the second or third time I'd ever heard him do that in half a century. I hear it from the kitchen, through the wooden shutters above the window box. The man is under unbelievable duress. But that's how much you have to worry about someone on Day Twenty-Three. I stay inside, quiet, no need to make a fuss. Everything will sort itself out. Extra fretting will not help. They trundle into the kitchen, where I greet Linda at arm's length. Full immune-deficiency protocol. Everything has been cleaned with Lysol wipes. Countertops, chairs, doorknobs, window latches, faucets. Floors scrubbed, dust eliminated, windows shut. "Welcome home, Linda," I say.

She smiles. What a long, strange trip it's been.

TAKING MY SEAT
Los Angeles
November 2017

We move slowly from the dining room to the living room. The hardwood floor creaks as our weight shifts, releasing the faint scent of Murphy Oil Soap. One of the framed pieces on the mauve-painted wall is a well-preserved poster from our young-adult lives, depicting a wild and joyous New Orleans at the height of Mardi Gras. We went there together for a week of music and food in 1983 and developed a lifelong devotion to the New Orleans Saints. Today we're just headed to the living room, where Linda sits on the cream-colored couch under the curtained double windows looking out onto the old neighborhood that grew with the movie industry in the late 1920s. A little afternoon light dribbles onto the glass table. I take one of the deep leather club chairs, and we settle in for a game of chess.

During this visit, I am taking an online course with my Zen friend. He broadcasts a talk on Wednesday evenings, followed by discussion with callers. The course is called Taking the One Seat and focuses on personal autonomy. In Zen they don't think that there is any sort of separate entity within you. There's no notion of a soul or self. They think there exists a single empty fullness, or full emptiness, that experiences itself as all our different temporary, sentient streams. That experience at any moment in any stream anywhere might be called soul, right there, boom—a moment of experiencing. That's all perfectly clear and fine. In Zen they say it gets messy only because the individual mind gets a false notion of itself—a self-concept. But of course we all have a self-concept, and we must, to be functional people.

"I" is a self-referential concept we use, so when you say, "Hey, Rikki," my system comes up with a social construct for you to interact with. It's an idea, but somehow, the way the self-reflective mind works (which I do not understand, but Doug Hofstadter offers a pretty interesting discussion in his book *I Am a Strange Loop*), we end up actually feeling like we truly *are* whatever concept we've got. Like we are a permanent entity, solid and real, with attributes and qualities and weaknesses and character. Like a soul. But in Zen, I'm considered just whatever it is to be aware at this moment. (The whole mystery is in the word "aware." What is that, experientially?)

They say in Buddhism that the locus of suffering is where your self-concept doesn't match up with reality. Here's what I'm thinking: My self-concept is a little twisted because of a rocky preverbal start. The more I untwist it so it reflects what I'm really like as a human being, the less conflicted I will feel.

It's Zen, so there's a paradox: If there is no individual in the stream, who takes the one seat? Who is trying to be autonomous? Spiritual teachers never answer this question, but I think some make it harder than it needs to be. The point is to experience yourself as you are as a human being, whatever that is, without the curtain of the self-concept blocking or coloring the experience. I've found many different meditation and contemplative practices in the yoga and Zen traditions that help to train my mind so it can begin to see without the lens of the self-concept.

In this class, I think we're talking about ways we can bring something into the world from our rich inner storehouse, getting it past the self-concept mechanism without distortion. Not unlike, I consider, trying to do abstract expressionist painting. So there's an assumption: that the authentic human being and her storehouse of energy, beneath and before the self-concept got installed, are not only accessible but worth accessing. There is an assumption that they are good, useful, beneficial, or healing in some way.

I have been confused about this for a long time. Sometimes my agitated feelings have seemed wild, angry, disruptive, or hostile. I have often feared my "core" self is not very good. At other times, my emotions are more positive and stable: compassionate, courageous, or confident. What is the real me?

In Buddhism, at least my American interpretation of it, the essence of what I am as a human being is considered good. It is a repository of confidence, generosity, and inclusiveness. It generates qualities I need when I need them, such as courage, wisdom, or kindness. This is quite a different notion than that of a sinful soul. There is no sinful soul in this view—just a rich, full being experiencing some confusion as it takes form; specifically, my form.

In the class we are looking at values from the repository that we aspire to manifest in our lives. What values really matter to me and tend to dominate my choices? I'm looking at what I actually value based on how I behave. I always want to get real, be authentic, speak truth, and drop appearances. I'm never satisfied with half-truths or the surface picture. Authenticity is clearly one of my values. The proposal is to look more deeply at what that means to me. What does it mean to get to the bone? Thinking about delusions, I am willing to get to the bone—even the marrow—if that is what it takes to clear delusions and awaken awareness in ever deeper layers.

Journaling about living values, I unexpectedly discover trust to be a core feature in my strategies for living. Trust is so close to faith that I cringe to think it could be a value I hold deeply. I eschew belief in favor of open curiosity and questioning. I find that beliefs get in the way of deep investigation. But *trust*. It's true that I deeply trust life. I trust that life is doing something, and that we individually are doing something in life. Personally, I need the comfort that trust brings to offset authenticity, because sometimes truth is hard to bear. I need to trust that it is worth it to keep moving through stories, healing and discarding them.

Much of my work here with Linda and Rick this week is to authentically trust life. In AA they have a slogan for it: "Let go and let God." I have my agenda for Linda's survival, but, at the same time, I have to honestly let go and trust what life is doing. There's what I want versus how life is, and there's me wanting to be present with both. I have a hard time with this.

We play chess on our iPads, using our multiplayer online chess game. We have learned and improved at about the same rate, so we keep each other challenged. Linda uses a standard opening that I'm used to. We tend to struggle for control of the four central squares at the opening of every game. When one of us strikes out in a new direction, she is taking a risk. Who knows what terrors lurk that we have not understood? How much farther a bishop may reach than you might imagine in the cheerful quiet of your neighborhood. How risky to let your knight linger while your queen moves out into the thick of things.

Now Linda sends a knight crashing into my front yard. I did not see that coming. I made sure I had pawns covering all the center squares. I lined up my bishop to attack one knight. My king was safely tucked away already. Suddenly, I've got her knight at my throat. Specifically, it's forking my two rooks. I have nothing to challenge that knight with. All my pieces are crowding the space, but none can take her piece. I am doomed to lose a rook. She will lose the knight, of course. I will take it with my other rook, whichever survives her stealthy strike. But Linda will be up two points in the body count.

Chess is a violent sport. You think about how to attack, how to deceive, how to decimate. If you succeed in entering enemy territory, you witness the devastation with pleasure. You cannot think in terms of mercy; you are being bombarded as well at every moment. My best strategy is to keep her on her back foot while whacking away at her defenses, make aggressive moves so she has to defend, and challenge pieces that she defends with. I think about whether to lose. How are Linda's spirits today? Would a defeat undo her, leaving her too discouraged to go on? But she surprised me with that knight and then a sudden, sweeping queen drive.

Linda takes a game as a game. She can take it, win or lose. When we were kids, she always knew more, was smarter, could win at everything. I would cheat whenever possible to give myself some slight advantage, but our twenty-six-month age difference defeated me. I would pout. Parcheesi, Clue, Sorry. I was always slamming my cards or dice or "man" down in frustration. These days, I go through cycles when I play chess with Linda. I run the gamut from willing to lose and willing to destroy her. For me, a game is rarely just a game.

These are the things I think about: Is she drinking enough fluid? Did anyone wipe down that coaster? How is she feeling? Can she swallow any food now? Is she afraid of death? Has she finished grieving the loss of hair, strength, and lung capacity, or does it sneak up on her when she's tying a shoelace? Would she share her grief if it came up?

We talk about Mommy's death, the guilt and shame that linger, Mommy's loss of power over the years. We try to make sense of it. We try to see if we have any harmful tendencies like Mommy's, and we are both sure we have counteracted any such thing. I have worked with gobs of self-pity over recent years. My weapon is responsibility. I try to take 100 percent responsibility for what is happening in my life. If X is happening to me, what am I doing to create that, or encourage that, or create an atmosphere where that is okay?

For example, my own self-deprecating attitude could invite people to dismiss me, which could then trigger self-pity in me. There's a cycle here, a tit for tat. I have been complicit in setting up situations where I've ended up a victim or felt sorry for myself. It's subtle, too. I doubt people think of me as a victim type. But I now understand how an unconscious pattern drives this behavior. I diminish myself before you do; then, when I feel diminished, that proves I was at risk. It's a vicious cycle. The way out for me is thinking in terms of 100 percent ownership. I am the one who has to grapple with the situations that appear in my form, both body and mind. Who else can deal with them for me?

On the other hand, you can take this responsibility thing too far the wrong way if you are conflict-averse. You can use it to avoid punching people when the situation calls for a straight right. I have a way of taking on too much responsibility beyond what is mine to take. If we go to the beach and you decide you don't want to carry a jacket and you get cold, I tend to think I should give you my jacket. This leads to my letting people treat me disrespectfully, because it must be my fault if you do. This bent way of thinking took me down some dark paths when I used it to let other people get away with shit. So I have to take ownership of that twist on ownership, too.

Nowadays I can slow down to see how and when I turn on the victim attitude. It happens sometimes when Jill and I get into a disagreement. Jill will be expressing her experience (which feels to me like yelling), and I hit that place in me that collapses, like Mother running out of rope. Instead of standing up for myself, I might just feel hurt. From there, things go south; my victim consciousness does no one any good. I feel hurt; I project blame; Jill feels accused and defends herself. I feel rejection and get hurt more.

But when I can see it happen, then I have a place to stand. I can get into my witness stance. I can stop the train at "I feel hurt." That becomes, "I am aware of hurt feelings. These are difficult to feel."

The second voice, that of a witness, has a stance from which she can observe what arises without judgment or control. "I am free of unconscious patterns that undermine my power," I try saying out loud to myself in the bathroom mirror. I can hear that it is not true, yet. I see the authentic face of an earnest person trusting the process. She has a strong intention.

The time finally comes to face the intimidating Pill Tray. Rick ordered two pillboxes. The smaller box will hold the midday pills. The larger box provides slots for seven days a week, a.m. and p.m. We have eighteen different pills in various shapes and sizes. Multiple pills are taken multiple times a day. Some are taken every day, some once or twice a week. One is a patch; one is to be taken for symptoms of rash, or another for symptoms of nausea, or another for sleep. Medicines for episodic symptoms do not go in the main Pill Tray.

I make a grid on a fresh white sheet of paper, using a mechanical pencil with an eraser. I list each medicine, mark the time of day; the number of pills; and the shape, color, and size of each pill. I revise this several times. In my final version, I leave space to note the latest changes doctors and nurses have phoned in. Medication is, we know now, a magical art. Every contingency is covered. Nevertheless, in coming weeks the dosages will get mixed up and the wrong number of some pills will get taken. Symptoms will get exacerbated, and doctors will be clueless—until Linda realizes the mix-up. And that too shall pass.

Rick and I make dinners each evening, and we all settle in to watch a show and eat on TV trays. I recall with gloom our childhood TV trays, whose TV dinners saved many meals from disaster. Mommy would deal with Daddy in a different room. She could get us in front of the TV before he got home. She never knew in what condition—or, for that matter, what time or whether—he'd arrive.

If Daddy had too many martinis before Mommy fed him dinner, our evening would go to hell. Daddy's rampages began as a slow grumble. I can't hear the words in my memory, just the danger signal burning. Was he drunk already? How did it play out? "Dick, just eat," Mother would beg. "Here, eat this. Here's another drink, Dick, don't. . ." What would he say? How did it devolve so quickly?

"You bitch, don't you attack me. I don't have to take shit from you, you fu . . ." I couldn't discern from the living room his frightening, alien voice. I couldn't hear, I didn't remember, I didn't want to know the confusion of mean and dirty words my father slung at my mother.

"Dick, stop. The children. Please keep your voice down . . ." Always the edge of fear, panic, never the sound of assertive power, never the sound of strength. The sound of escalation. Then Mommy was pushing us into the den with the TV and Daddy was trundling into the other room, with the wet bar, where he would trade the martini, already too warm, for scotch on the rocks. Shouting from there. Whispers. The voices more energized and ugly.

You had to get Daddy to eat before he started drinking. This was Mommy's job, but Mommy couldn't keep a horse from drinking water. She was powerless over the situation, so she dumped it on us, especially Linda. Linda was smarter than Mommy; that's why she went to boarding school. She was not going to spend her life in this quagmire.

Even when she's home for vacation, she takes it on the chin. One year when we are living in LA, we try a family trip to a favorite desert oasis.

Spring 1965

The drive to Palm Springs from LA took about a million hours, with three jerky kids in the backseat and two adults engulfed in a scary love-hate saga sitting in the front. We played a find-it spelling game to pass the time. Linda had just found a *J* on a license plate, and I was pouting for lack of a *K*. Beth was probably reading; maybe she played the spelling game, too, and I helped her. I would have helped Bethy to spite Linda. Traffic on the I-10 East was gridlocked during spring break, and my mother was already bitching at Daddy and making him edgy. She reached back and found someone's leg with her fingers, grabbing and pinching hard. "Stop arguing back there," she said again.

"Listen to your mother," Daddy commanded. Everyone was getting too hungry, and we were all ready to kill each other hours before we arrived. Even Bethy, at six, knew the family pattern. Things were going to blow.

Blowing meant shouting and tears, sometimes a punch or a broken vase. Mom always came unglued; Daddy's viciousness and threats of violence brought her down completely. I wonder, were there no resources for wealthy white women in the white suburbs of Chicago or, later, of Los Angeles? She had no context for dealing with this; her father drank beer with buddies on the corner and came home singing. He died young, after surviving World War I in a Russian prison camp and walking home to Austria after the war. He was not an unbalanced man. Daddy must have confused Mother beyond her means. She learned to match him drink for drink, leaving us on our own.

In Palm Springs, she was desperate to supply dinner before he got violent. For some reason, we had booze with us but not food. As soon as we arrived, Mom sent Linda out with the car to a deli to get sandwiches. Bethy and I loaded into the car with Linda. Far safer with her. It was like a desperado raid. There was no time; it was all a rush before Daddy killed something. Why couldn't he just have a Snickers bar and chill?

We cruised out onto the desert Highway 118, back toward the shops and restaurants on Highway 111. Things were vast and spread out down here, in the dry, low hills below the San Jacinto Mountains. But the goddamn deli was closed. We were six, thirteen, and sixteen years old, and we were going to find some corned beef sandwiches for the wacked-out drunks back at the vacation pad if it killed us. We headed over to Bob Hope Drive and scanned the highway, trying to find something Linda thought would fit the bill. It was too late at night; the stores had closed at sundown.

Eventually we got something unworthy at a late-night grocery. Traipsing back to the hotel, we found the parents in a Sad State. Daddy was drunk and yelling; Mommy was hysterical and crying. She blamed Linda for Daddy's drunkenness. Linda just stood there, staring at them. I went outside and stuck a kitchen knife in a tree. Bethy found a corner to set up her bed and read. No one had dinner. Daddy passed out in a chair by the pool and was still there in the morning.

Tonight, Rick and I make a small portion for Linda. She can't eat much; she's been nauseated since Day Zero, and it won't let up until near Day Ninety. It doesn't appear to be GVH, though. In fact, we have no signs of GVH. Nausea is probably from the cocktail of drugs.

My checklist is astonishing. Linda is a poster child for allogeneic stem cell transplants. Things are progressing slowly and on target:

- Viable donor

- Perfect match

- Get into trial to stay alive until transplant

- Complete trial

- Get transplant

- Transplant takes over 93 percent—TBD after thirty-day biopsy (so far so good)

- No graft versus host (GVH) disease!

- Heal (so far so good)

- Kill tumors (we have to wait for a six-month post-transplant PET scan)

MARROW BIOPSY

Duarte
November 2017

Linda and I ride out to City of Hope to get a bone marrow biopsy. She sleeps in the car, dozing to my playlist of great rock from our college years at UC Santa Barbara: Van Morrison, Tom Petty, Paul Simon. We were at UCSB together for a year, I as a freshman living on campus and Linda as an upperclassman in an apartment on the beach. Linda took her first year at the Jesuit school Creighton University in Omaha. Our family moved from Chicago to Los Angeles after her freshman year, so she joined us in California and transferred to UCSB while I finished high school and Elizabeth was still in grammar school.

In the summer of 1968, I went up to Santa Barbara for a year. After that year, Rick, Linda, another friend, and I migrated north to California's political action center, the San Francisco Bay Area, including Berkeley and Oakland. After a year, Rick and Linda returned and launched their married life together, but I stayed. Silicon Valley was not here yet; in 1969, it was still just the Menlo Park investors, Lockheed, Fairchild, a nascent Intel, and the four-node ARPANET.

Today I navigate the lattice of LA freeways and arrive at the Cope's valet parking without a hitch. But Linda objects. "No, no, go ahead and park. The walk is good for me." Bless her soul. Her lungs are still messed up; she can't get enough oxygen to move beyond a plod. So we park and Linda gets out a mask and wraps the loops around her ears, stretching the cotton over her mouth and nose. We walk, slowly, no problem. A jitney whizzes over to offer a ride, but we decline. The driver nods and smiles. He is proud of Linda for walking. Patients in recovery need to walk, but it's harder than we non-patients can understand. Their blood chemistry is imbalanced; they've taken poisonous chemicals; their hair has fallen out. We walk along, feeling pretty sparky. Linda is making real time. She uses a cane to steady herself.

We go past the Spirit of Life fountain, and I remember the dread and hope that flooded me the first time I came here to get the slew of tests and exams to qualify as a donor. I recall the exuberance and hope that intoxicated me after the abundant stem cell extraction session. We have been through so much together.

Once we are indoors, Linda can remove the mask. Masks are mostly useful for big stuff floating around outside: fungi and bugs and pollen-y things. Viruses can pass through the mask. We have to stay away from airborne viruses. Airborne viruses are forbidden in City of Hope. We wander down some corridors and take an elevator. We use the sanitizer after touching buttons.

We have to go up to the clinic to get a blood test. Linda is being closely monitored. She will come to City of Hope twice a week for weeks. Eventually she will go down to once a month. That seems years from today. Today we need to assess all the blood chemistry: RBC, WBC, electrolytes, neutrophils, creatinine, hemoglobin. She verifies her name, her patient number, her doctor. She gets weighed. She rates her pain and discomfort so they can catch anything before it's a problem. She has low pain. The nurse takes her temperature and measures her blood pressure, then takes the blood sample. We sanitize and ambulate through the buildings to the lab where they will do the bone marrow biopsy.

Linda is nervous about this procedure because it is painful and uncomfortable. She has to lie on her stomach while the doctor fathoms the skin and hipbone with a thickish needle. It reminds me of the needle used in the amniocentesis they did when I was pregnant. But this needle aspirates bits of bone and marrow from the inside of Linda's hipbone. And she is in luck. A nurse practitioner, NP—not a doctor—is going to perform the procedure. Nurses, Linda has observed, are much more likely to have the gentle touch, the patience, and the ability to listen that makes a biopsy nearly painless and hardly stressful.

A second nurse will assist. She has taken packets, tubes, and instruments from a kit she has brought in. I am peering around her shoulder, trying not to take up any space. The nurses murmur to each other, the assistant picking up a this or a that and asking about its use. Does she not know how to do this procedure?

"Are you in training for this procedure?" I ask, with what I hope is a disarming smile.

The NP answers for the supposed trainee. "Each lab is slightly different. We just go over the procedure each time." They go back to each other. Finally, the assisting nurse turns to Linda and positions her on the table. The NP takes up a smaller needle and pulls it from its protective sleeve.

"Each doctor—or nurse practitioner—does it their own way. Some aspirate the bone first, some last," says the assisting nurse. She reaches over Linda's back to hold something for the NP, who begins talking to Linda.

"First, we anesthetize the area. You will feel this." She injects the anesthetic.

While they wait for that to kick in, the NP explains to Linda what happens next. She pulls the larger needle from its protective wrap. She positions it above Linda's hipbone.

"You will feel some pressure now," she says, as she strong-arms the needle, but with a steady, firm push, not a shove. The point goes in smoothly. No sound from Linda. "Okay?"

"Yes."

It takes a few minutes, and Linda cannot move while the needle is in. It chips the bone, sucking up the clip for analysis. The needle bears down through bone into marrow and vacuums out a good scoop. Talking as she works, the NP explains what will happen next, where Linda will feel pressure, what the sounds are. This is all done by hand. Linda appears relaxed, asking short questions as they proceed. She tells me later that she got through this the way she gets through all these procedures—by focusing on exactly what is happening and asking questions to make sure she is not missing anything. This 100 percent here-for-it technique, she assures me, works for other things, too.

"What will you do for Thanksgiving?" the NP asks, as she strips the latex off her gloved hands.

"Well, since I'm immune-compromised, obviously, we'll just be staying home together. No big dinner this year." Linda, still lying facedown, sounds a little wistful. I thought she would be relieved, but it makes sense that she would be sad about another thing that cancer is taking from her. I just hope this time it's not cancer. It's recovery from a transplant. I hope. We won't know about cancer until the six-month PET.

Linda's survival is still in the hopeful statistical range; she's not out of the woods yet. This biopsy will tell us a lot. The assistant says what we all hope. "Next year, you can celebrate all you want. This year, it's better to rest."

This biopsy will tell us the degree to which the implant has taken root. The doctor wants to see 93 percent of the bone marrow showing the new genetics. Cancerous cells should be rare in the marrow. We want the vast preponderance of bone marrow to be produced from the 6.5 million pluripotent stem cells per kilogram that they infused into Linda thirty-two days ago. We will know in about a week.

DAY THIRTY-SIX: THANKSGIVING

Los Angeles
November 2017

I was planning to stay a week and drive home Wednesday. But Thursday is Thanksgiving, and they have not made any arrangements. Their son, Ari, lives a few miles away, on the other side of the 405 traffic barrier, and can easily join them. The annual custom is for Linda to cook a traditional meal and invite Rick's side of the family. This year, Linda is free of the burden but no replacement plans have been made.

Growing up in the suburbs outside Chicago in the 1950s and '60s, we gathered at Aunt Margaret's, the most centralized location, with a big kitchen. Mom had the biggest house, but Auntie M. had the biggest kitchen. The women would congregate around Margaret's round wooden table with its green-painted, square-backed doweled chairs. The men, in the living room, drank beer and watched sports and shouted at each other. All the women would bring dishes for the table. We always brought pearled onions and scalloped potatoes. Looking back, I really think the men just brought beer, even my unmarried uncles, who came and ate the most. We women would buy the ingredients, prepare the food, heat the food, polish the silver, set the tables (we had two—the grownups' table and the kids' table), serve the food, clear the tables, pack the food, and do the dishes. The men ate and enjoyed the family holiday. I wonder why it took me so many years to notice.

Thanksgiving 1962

My father drank scotch—Dewar's White—and that led to rapid decay, even with the padding and dilution from a big dinner. Uncle Ray had the Pat Boone Thanksgiving show going in the recreation room downstairs for the kids.

We kids were going through a knock-knock-joke phase.

Knock, knock.

Who's there?

Canoe.

Canoe who?

Canoe help me with my homework?

Har-de-har-har.

Then we got going with our puns. Tom Swifties were the hot ones of the day.

"'Welcome to my tomb,' said Tom cryptically," said Joanne.

"No—'I'm going bald,' Tom *bawled*," I rejoined.

"No, you idiot, it's 'I'm losing my hair,'" Linda corrected.

Elizabeth tried, "You try to shut the door, but the door shuts you," but she was only just five a few weeks ago.

"'Let's help that sick bird,' said Tom ill-eagley," put in Little Ray.

While this was going on with the cousins, darker streams activated in my increasingly drunken father. Uncle Ray was trying to get Daddy under control. But Daddy had to tell his joke. We could hear Uncle Ray first: "Dick, stay up here!" The kids were downstairs, the adults upstairs in the living room. "Don't tell them that, Dick.

Stop!" And there was Daddy. Losing his balance on the first step, he lurched to his right and his shoulder caught the wall. An athlete, he bounced back to center and controlled the overcorrection by grabbing a banister. "I got one," he was shouting to us kids. He slid two steps and stabilized on the fourth. That was half the short flight of stairs; he was almost down, and then he was able to grab the curve of the countertop at the bottom. "I got one," he slurred.

"Dick, come back here." Aunt Margaret's voice, angry now.

"'I'm coming, Mother,' Oedipus ejaculated." He laughed.

We were stunned. Each kid was wondering what the words meant. Uncle Ray was embarrassed and couldn't look at us. I knew the word *Oedipus*—that was Greek; I remembered it from my prince training. I was suspicious about *ejaculated*. I was pretty sure it was a bad word about a secret thing.

"It's a pun!" Daddy insisted.

The kids knew to be embarrassed for Uncle Dick, as this was not the first time, but at least he was telling a joke, instead of insulting someone or yelling or saying dirty things. Although this might have been dirty. We were not even teenagers yet, except for Linda. We did the fake laugh—*pretty funny, Uncle Dick*—and waited for Uncle Ray to get him back with the grown-ups.

I call Jill. "I think I should stay and have Thanksgiving dinner with them. We really have something to be grateful for this year, so we should arrange something for the four of us."

"Yes, baby, you should," Jill says. "That would be good. You guys should celebrate together. We can Skype you from my brother's house. Order stuff from Whole Foods."

We order from Gelson's. Everyone thinks this is a great idea. We can gather and eat traditional foods and celebrate in our own, quiet way. Since I'm a vegetarian, I make sure there are dishes for me. As a good codependent, I don't want everyone to sit down to dinner only to discover I can eat nothing but salad. Everyone would feel bad. I briefly think I am so tired that I am not even aware of what I might want to eat. What mostly matters to me is having a warm, restorative family evening, without unconscious patterns. Ha! An evening of freedom!

Ari comes and brings Rick's favorite pie. Linda eats enough to stuff a hummingbird, bless her, but Rick, Ari, and I have roasted sweet potatoes and gelled cranberries and sautéed spinach, and the guys have Cornish game hens. Afterward, we plan to watch a movie, as was their family tradition after guests left on previous Thanksgivings. But, blessing of blessings, this year we migrate instead to the living room, where Rick's guitar waits in its stand.

When we were all in college, long before any Aris were conceived, we used to sit up nights and drink cheap red Gallo wine and sing the blues. Or any Dylan song; Rick is a Dylan guy. Here, at our Thanksgiving, we four represent more than sixty-five years of Linda's life. Her sister, her husband, her firstborn. Rick has been with Linda for something like forty-five years. There are dozens of songs we have sung and celebrated in various configurations of family and friends over the years: songs from Ari's childhood, when he was the baby; songs from Rick's childhood, when he was the baby. We all four sing, even Linda, whose vocal cords sustained long-term damage in the bombing raids. We all sing like little angels, harmonies and disharmonies alike.

This is the Thanksgiving celebration we really needed.

RECOVERY

THE PANIC ATTACK
Santa Cruz Mountains
November 2017

Traffic is light up Interstate 5. I plow up the Central Valley, past the 18-wheelers and holiday travelers, to Pacheco Pass west without stopping to eat. The car skippers up 101 and 85 until I ascend Highway 17 onto the ridge of the Santa Cruz Mountains. That's where you start to feel like you're escaping the hectic life of the valley. Redwoods and eucalyptus line the winding route up the hill. When I first came to the Bay Area and joined the student demonstrations at UC Berkeley in 1969, this was a two-lane road with no center divider. The serpentine mountain pass today is a four-lane, divided, well-banked highway. We have only one overpass from Los Gatos to Scotts Valley, and we should have two or three. But the one we have is the one I need, at Summit Road. I get off and head east by south.

Another ten miles curve up forested mountain routes before I come to our private road. A round of robins swoops across my path, trying to lure me away from their nests. I cruise on past their tiny roosts. Home!

I lug all my gear out of the car and into the right rooms: kitchen, bedroom, office, laundry. If I am not too done in after a trip, I like to unpack and get all my stuff back where it goes. Today I am done in. I just leave all the stuff out, ready to be dealt with in the morning by a refreshed version of me. I am longing for a shower in my own bathroom. I can start to really wind down. The transplant's done, and it's working. I behaved myself commendably, and it seems like the effect of quiet concentration has been similar to being on retreat. My mind feels balanced and able to focus.

The skin on my back has been itchy and sensitive this past week; now, I find two unexpected bumps where I scratched between my angel bones. I am weary, a little crabby, and abruptly, unexpectedly, now thinking about skin cancer. *Shit. Shit, shit, shit. Stop thinking that.* How many years have I meditated, put all together? Maybe twenty-five, in the fifty years since High-School Rikki got a mantra from the Maharishi Mahesh Yogi organization. Twenty-five years' worth of sitting on my butt, noticing the activity of my mind. Developing a capacity to witness with kindness. Yet today I can't stop obsessing about one little thought running around in my head like a puppy with a bone. And it is making me hop around frantically, instead of taking a relaxing shower.

I want to get a good look at my back. I shuffle over to the bathroom mirror and pretzel, to little avail. Grabbing a hand mirror, I sit near a window with good natural light. Okay, this is nothing, I see, just dry skin. But I can't see the second area. I am frustrated; I am upset. Abruptly, I am very upset. My face starts to heat up; my chest catches on fire. All the feelings in my mind collapse into a funnel inside me and sink down into a vortex somewhere behind my solar plexus. I hear myself sucking for air. *It's a fucking Dementor,* I think. Breath comes after a couple jerky pulls. *I have got to get out of here. I'm panicking.*

I get out of there and go into the bedroom and sit down on the couch under the window to do breathing exercises, but I can't remember how to do them. I can count, so I count. I close my eyes and put my head in my hands and count breaths, one, two, three. Good. One, two, three again. Good. I begin some simple yoga breathing to calm my mind. I do this by imagining that my in-breath draws the air up the spinal column, from the base of the spine to the head. As I breathe in, I picture my breath rising up my spine like mercury in a thermometer or water in a straw. When I exhale, I relax and picture the breath running back down the spinal channel. Breathing in makes breath rise to the forehead; breathing out makes breath fall to the tailbone.

What happened in there? I ask myself later, with a ceramic mug of chamomile tea in my hand. *I panicked*, I answer myself. I wasn't expecting it, but I just went over an edge without much warning. Sweat dripped down my forehead. My vision tunneled. I had a desperate, screaming feeling around my heart. What's going on with me? It makes sense that thoughts of cancer are distressing. But, as it's turning out, the stem cell treatment is working and all signs are positive. This is a great moment. It is *the* moment. Why am I celebrating with a panic attack?

Some memories seem innocent, like bells that jingle in the wind. Some memories cramp the future they live in and the filters you can see through. They create the questions you chase and the pains you're always trying to soothe. I have black-and-white images of my father. He was the hero at high noon and the madness in the dark. Daddy had a great, scary *bwa-ha-ha* laugh that he would use, upon request, to scare us in the basement. *Bwa-ha-ha* was fun because then Daddy was just pretending. When he was drunk, he was Unpredictable and sometimes hurt himself. Good things never happened without a bad thing following, like a stomachache after too many grapes off the vine in spring. You always felt like he lived on an edge.

In our childhood home, his antique mahogany chest of drawers stood just to the right of the doorway into their bedroom. Its private surface was above my head, but I could see the glimmer of his special things. His wallet, keys, and money folded into a small clip. I used to sneak five-dollar bills from it. A small black plastic comb. And, in the top right-hand drawer, under a folded, ironed white handkerchief, his nine-millimeter German P08 Luger pistol, a black trophy of his nightmarish wartime in Germany. I touched its frightening, hard edges. This was from the scary place where Daddy went before we were born. A German soldier had it. Did Daddy kill him? Was it loaded? It was a symbol to me of Daddy's mysterious maleness, which impelled and empowered him to go into an exotic world of violence and foreign lands. It had to do with his nightmares and things I did not know about, adventures and frightening human dramas beyond my reach. I never held that pistol in my hand. I was terrified of it, that its darkness would leak into me and make me shoot it. I worried about my father's stability. In eight-year-old terms, I thought, *My father needs a mother.* But Mommy was already at the end of her rope. Later on, I knew I had to keep things like guns away from Daddy. It was always there, the risk of someone getting hurt, in the dresser drawer or the kitchen cabinet or the garage.

There's an explosively dangerous energy hulking just inside me now, and I feel like the wrong train of thought can set it off. It's not exactly the fear of cancer; rather the panic rises at the thought (shiver) that I can't *see* part of me. Because I am trying not to have that train of thought, it starts on its own. I discover that I can't see my own head, inside my mouth, or, for that matter, anywhere inside my body. And, yes, these thoughts trigger a froth of the panic, so I quickly pull my attention away, like a finger from a hot stove. I don't even want to risk thinking about why that sort of idea bothers me. It's about loss of control, it's about the unknown, and that's all I know.

Here I am, having panic, with a dark, despairing creature grabbing me on the inside of my throat in the quiet of my own home, on a day I could be celebrating. I don't want to think of the darkness in Daddy's mind. I don't want to harm myself. I don't want to get depressed again. *Oh please don't be that depression please don't come for me please go away please let me get through this please be all right.*

Have I been using silence to cut myself off from the energy that lifts mountains? If so, maybe it's a good thing to have a panic attack. Maybe that will get me to refocus. Sometimes the wrong train can get you to the right station.

HELP FROM THE 90 PERCENT

Santa Cruz Mountains
November 2017

They say that only a small percentage, perhaps 5 percent, of a brain's resources contribute to normal waking awareness. The other 95 percent is doing Everything Else. Maybe those percentages are off, but that's not the point. Make it 90/10 percent for discussion's sake.

I'm thinking that some of my 90 percent arranged to have a panic attack so I'd pay attention. I've been ignoring things; I've been pushing too much down and out of consciousness, including a lot of grief I held but hadn't released. I could use some of the 90 percent to process grief. Heck, I could use it to improve my strike accuracy. I count on my inner world to support me, to organize my energy toward fulfilling my intentions. I hope it's sending me a panic attack for a good reason, but I'm a little frightened of myself.

The first thing is to see a dermatologist and rule out cancer. I call for the appointment and can get in next week. My next priority is to avoid a recurrence of panic. I could easily get into a panic about panic. Later on, I will think about this. When I feel fear, it might be that I am mostly afraid of more fear, and that would be a useful thing to know. But right now, I am afraid of this energy. Panicky trains of thought flicker at the edge of my attention like flames flickering on the Loma Prieta ridge. I'm grinding my teeth. So, second thing, I put in calls to psychiatrists in the Los Gatos medical group.

I want one of the "-azepams"—lorazepam, clonazepam—benzo-diazepines with fast-acting sedative effects. These things really calm anxiousness quickly, but they're extremely addictive. For someone who really never could keep a half bottle of wine in the house—I always finished it—having this drug around means having a relation-ship with it. I will count the number of pills I have, break them in half, avoid using them as long as possible, dish them out attentively, all just to be sure I still have a handful in case I need them.

The panic attack continues to resonate, causing general dis-quiet and clutches of anxiousness. That and the looming monster of decade-old depression really light a fire under me. I do not want that darkness taking control again. I'm not sure I understand how I got out of it before. Could I just sweep it under the rug and give it time? Get over to the gym and work it out on the bag or sparring with Dawn? The thing is, though, sweeping it under the rug doesn't align with my intention. I vowed to walk through every wisdom gate, and here's a gate into something I need to explore. What's trying to get my attention, and how can I learn to listen to it?

This time, I am willing to reach out for help, but what kind of help do I need? I want to explore this, not just make it go away. At the level of the body, I can see the dermatologist, get drugs from the psychiatrist, and work out. But what can I do differently to restore mental balance? Third thing: I call a friend of mine who is a teacher of yoga and ask her about breathing techniques. She reminds me of sev-eral that I learned at the yoga center. In particular, she recommends long-exhale breathing. This promotes a sense of balance, peace, and ease after several rounds of breath. I add this to my meditation practice, but it is also easy to do on the spot without being obvious.

At the level of spirit, do I need support from a spiritual advisor? I think what I really need is simply spiritual friendship. Fourth thing: I call my friends Jan and Illana, who practice Zen. They have two dogs, Woody and Cookie, and at this time in our friendship they live in Aptos, near the beach. Woody and Zoey are friends, so the four of us humans arrange to get together for a meal and a walk with our three dogs along Monterey Bay.

"How's your sister?" Jan asks, as Woody, a full-size adult male poodle, drags her down the sidewalk. We are walking the few blocks from their home to the beach. Jill and Illana are walking behind us with Zoey and Cookie on leashes.

"Amazing, Jan." I go over some of the statistics and Linda's status. "But, strangely, I'm kind of unraveling. Instead of celebrating. It's weird."

Jan pulls back on Woody, who likes to be in front of the pack. Jan used to be the head coach of the women's tennis team at UC Berkeley, my alma mater. She takes a pragmatic approach to things. "But it makes sense, unraveling after you went through this whole thing with her," she says. "I'd be exhausted."

"Yes," I admit.

"I know when I go through something with family, sisters especially, it can be really difficult. Do you feel healing between you two as sisters?" Jan asks.

When we get to the sand, the dogs are eager, but we keep them on leash until we are clear of people.

"I do, Jan. You just go past all the pettiness and get down to what really matters."

"Maybe you're doing some purging and cleansing. Getting it out of your system." Illana and Jill let the dogs go, and they race past us. Jan pulls Woody hard to get him to sit, then quickly clicks his leash off, and he races to join Cookie and Zoey.

"That's a good point," I say.

Illana has picked up a stick and is throwing it for Woody to chase. He chases it into the water, but he won't swim after it. Zoey chases Woody, not the stick.

"And then you will be free to create something new, like that Zen story about the stone woman who gives birth to a child at night," she adds.

"How so?" I ask. My first reaction to everything in Zen is a clenched bewilderment. I'm always afraid I won't get it.

"Like you had this freezing in your relationship, but in the dark, where you can't see, the silence was busy giving birth to something new and beautiful."

It's so good to have friends. We run down to the water and take our shoes off and walk in the cold, fresh sea.

At the level of psyche, would I benefit from counseling with a therapist? What would you ask for from a mental-health switchboard? It's a long story, and I'm not sure I know what's going on. How long would it take to build the trust and relationship you need to investigate this sort of thing? Decades ago, when I was just getting sober, I had a great support system for clearing my head. I could to go to a meeting, call a sponsor, talk with my therapist, or have dinner with an AA friend.

I say "just getting sober" as if this were as simple as learning to drive or to speak traveler's French. It was not. Alcohol gave me a lot of relief and freedom. As a teen, I fell effortlessly into drinking. I had my first beer at the age of thirteen, at a party on a fall night in Northbrook, Illinois, where I first met Jackie Peterson and, later, Lou Stauffer. If memory serves, that beer morphed into shots of Stolichnaya from the bottle in the upstairs bedroom of an entirely different house with three people who, I will say in my defense, became my best friends over the next year. I suppose Lou drove me home, perhaps in his 1964 navy-blue Chevy Impala with dual overhead cams and racing tires. I was still a virgin; he was a gentleman and soon my first boyfriend. Daily drinking started in college. For fifteen more years, my most provocative, interesting, and talkative self came out only when fueled by alcohol. Drunk, I yearned to belong, to love, to impress, to pick fights, to find a home, to give my self over to divine passions, to hide, to die, to travel everywhere, and to write poems of ecstasy and devotion. Sober, I was generally tight, confused, lonely, frightened, or angry. Sober, I yearned to find an opening for my life and to have a drink. Drunk, I often blacked out and awoke in unfamiliar places with dim goblins creeping around my memory. "Just getting sober" involved first of all disconnecting from alcohol, and then dealing with all the other stuff.

Dealing with the other stuff meant going to daily AA meetings. Then a sponsor, AA colleagues, and the 12 Steps And, in due course, therapy. My best friend, Texas Patty, introduced me to her therapist, JoAnn, who was an energetic icon in our recovery community. Tackling addiction directly in her practice, she used tools and insights from the 12 Steps to supplement the power of psychotherapy. To work with her, I had to commit to not drinking, to going to AA meetings, and to being willing to take care of my shit. We worked together for a few years. I dealt with a lot of shit.

In AA meeting rooms and coffeehouses and the therapy office, I found ways to see through my confusion back to myself. I had a poor view of what was unfolding; I was inside looking out. Compared with the hard-edged outer world of objects, the inner world is murky, like an underwater montage of passages and canals. The inner vision is a subtle, shifting mirage of images and impressions. Somewhere in this, I hoped there was something I could grab onto.

The fabric of my thoughts and feelings was like tangled twine. I had difficulty knowing the truth or sorting out my feelings. Therapy provided a map of the territory: the dynamics of family alcoholism and the confusion of addiction. It offered clarity, insight, and little picks to tease out warp from weft, to cull knots and snarls.

My work with therapy and the 12 Steps brought about big shifts in how I viewed myself in the world. I learned to discern the emotions I experienced. JoAnn would ask me to pick one: angry, sad, happy, or scared. Most of my feelings fell into one of these categories. I would concentrate like heck and take a wild guess: Sad? No, angry? At any one time, I could remember only three. The one I had forgotten was usually the one I was experiencing.

I learned I could take responsibility for the impact of my actions. I don't always have to be right. I learned that you can change how you relate both to yourself and to what arises within you. You don't have to be overcome by feelings that erupt from within; you can learn to observe and even comfort them. You don't have to accept a sense of yourself as broken or messed up or lacking. I began to sense myself differently as a result of that work. The sense of me-ness that arises amid the whirring and whizzing in the dense tissue of the brain is flexible, not static or permanent. You can get a warped self-concept from childhood, but you can work with it to get some of the dents out. So that's what I set out to do now.

How can I get my self-concept refurbished? What does intuition suggest? What feels like it could really help me move through all this?

I think of the person who helped me confront alcoholism in the first place. Though none of us drinks anymore, I am drenched in family alcoholism and dynamics. Might that therapist still be around?

I check online. Yes, she has an active presence as a mental-health professional. I hear myself exhale, relief flowing like fresh water. That feels right. So, fifth thing, I instant-message her, briefly explaining: I know it's been thirty-five years, but are you available? . . . Transplant . . . Panic . . .

"I'd be honored," she writes, barely twenty-four hours later, on a Sunday. I'm in her office Tuesday morning. That turns out to be exactly the support I need, and more than I looked for.

It's a case of being protected by the energy that lifts mountains.

My old attitude had been that you rarely get help when you need it. But now I'm thinking I was mistaken. How is it that the energy that lifts mountains has lifted and protected me? It's made sure I had the cells Linda needed when she needed them with the potency she needed. Now it has carried me to a safe place to work out this stuff in my head. The protective energies, my 90 percent, and my intention have successfully conspired to get me to an old friend whom I can trust to keep going with the work of awakening, without any delay.

The energy that lifts mountains is a metaphor, but also, energy actually lifts mountains. It's the energy of heat and pressure, but that is not different from the energy in sunlight or electricity. Energy changes forms but is never lost or created. Sunlight becomes the plant life that becomes all our food. Decayed, compacted plant and animal life become oil and coal, which are easily converted to electricity. The energy fueling this thought is extracted from food in my cells during everyday metabolism. That energy is the same as the chemical energy my neurons are using to send electric impulses and trigger synapses, to think these thoughts and tell my fingers to type these words.

We don't know what energy actually *is*, but scientists can measure it precisely. It is something that empowers the shape and movement of form, and it can get captured in many different forms. It hovers within the world as particles, light waves, gravity, chemical bonds, heat, and motion. Vast gobs of energy released deep within earth as hot gas, magma, pressure, heat, and gravity move mountains. Tiny spurts of energy released deep within the mitochondria of neurons move thoughts. It's the same energy. It is in a constant state of change and flux between my system and everything else.

The energy released in food metabolism in trillions of my body's cells is instantly captured in little packets for use in other metabolic pathways. My ability to experience anything, including being alive, is grounded in the ways in which these cells manage the energy and molecules from food.

From the Eastern perspective, Indian philosophy looks at food as fuel that feeds the cycles of life. Food energizes action (a disordered movement called *rajas*) that moves energy from a state of harmonized potential (an upward movement called *sattva*) to form (a downward movement called *tamas*) and back. This thinking holds that "being" exists and is expressed in the world with the qualities of existence (*sat*), knowing (*chit*), and embracing (*ananda*). It says that being gives rise to individuals; we are each a bit of "being" that took form in body and mind. Our natural shape—both body and mind—has the intelligence it needs within its own form, and that intelligence embraces everything that it encounters naturally. This is experienced as your own inherent vitality, wisdom, and kindness. These qualities are already there, within a person, when you let go and let your intuition guide you.

Whether you look from the East or from the West, it took billions of years to form me. The life pulsing in cells evolved and replicated and cooked for billions of years before finally producing me. I am its grandchild. I am its baby. Why would it not embrace and protect me?

BE HERE NOW

Santa Cruz Mountains
December 2017

JoAnn's office is off the beaten track in the rolling, wooded high-lands of the eastern slope of the Santa Cruz Mountains. The curving drive through the open woodlands gives my mind a few minutes to unwind. When I park the car on the side of the road, I can hear quail *chi-ca-go*-ing to each other in the scrub off to the side. I take a complete cleansing breath. The air has a chilly bite from a gently rising mist, as morning sunlight penetrates the copse on the hillside. I am wound up pretty tightly, but I exhale fully and shake my shoulders loose. The chatter of a male California thrasher singing like a mockingbird tells me I'm standing near a nest. We've had a mild season. Are birds nesting already? I feel the fresh air on my skin. Will therapy calm the dragon hovering over my left shoulder? I am hopeful.

The office is decorated with feminine warmth and a bit of whimsy. Pale yellow walls enclose a restful, safe space. I exhale and feel my jaw soften. There is a hot water dispenser, tea, and mugs, but I'm a bit too edgy to mess with that stuff. I sit down in one of the black bucket chairs. A cream-and-tan abstract of a mother cow with her calf hangs on the wall across from me. I close my eyes and start alternate-nostril breathing, beginning on the right side. I don't want to start a train of thought or worry. In-breath for four counts; hold for eight. Exhale for eight. Switch. I do about five rounds.

Though I have not seen JoAnn in more than thirty years, since before my daughter was born, we waste no time with formalities. When she opens the door of the waiting room, I recognize her immediately and the elapsed decades present no barrier. In the consulting room, I take a seat on the cushy couch with pillows and a box of Kleenex. She invites me to jump in, and I start my story. My mother, my sisters. My parents, my family. Me. Is there any other story?

"And then I had this panic thing. I've been doing all this good stuff with my family—we've saved my sister's life—but for some reason, instead of celebrating, I'm having panic attacks. Like, throat-closed, no-breath anxiety." I'm holding one of the pillows in my lap and flipping it over and over as I talk.

"But you saved her life?" JoAnn interjects, smiling incredulously with her bright blue eyes. "How?" she asks.

In fact, just today we got the results of the bone marrow biopsy. The graft of my stem cells has rooted successfully in Linda's marrow and is producing new red and white blood cells. The medical team wanted to see 93 percent new genetics, but we did better. I race through the story, leaving a trail of medical terms, dangling adjectives and unfastened references. Lymphoma, Muay Thai, worst nightmare, almost over, after Mom's death, help.

"Just now you found out?"

"Yes, Linda texted the results just as I was driving here. It's working. The new genetics are 99 percent. That means her bone marrow will make a new immune system with the new genetics. It means it worked." I tell this astonishing story with a voice that sounds flat to me. Where is the elation? Maybe I'm just burnt out.

"Tell me about this panic."

JoAnn sends me home with a thick book detailing lots of tools used in the cognitive behavioral therapy (CBT) approach to panic and anxiety. There are names and descriptions of things that happen to me and experiences of people who work through them. There are a lot of techniques, one for every sort of issue and temperament. In the next few months, I will discover that psychotherapy is a lot like Buddhist practice. You clear away delusions and distortions that block access to your whole self and its expression. To help do this, you turn up the volume on the delusions; you put yourself in a situation where they become harder to ignore. In Buddhist practice, you use meditation and your relationships with other Buddhists to discover how your reactive mind works. In therapy, you use the intensity of the relationship and the dialogue in a similar way, like a microscope. You're not discovering it just to discover it, either; you have to work to bring it into presence, let it be healed and released. You have to change behavior and thoughts. It's not easy, but I know I have landed in the right place and will grow through this.

Over the next weeks, I start to make connections in my psyche. This panicky part is familiar, an old feeling from childhood. The "grasping hands of dark despair" that I feel in a panic attack are similar to the grasping hands that grew out of the dark walls in the hallways of the house in Northbrook where I sat to escape the monsters under the bed, but I couldn't lean against the walls because the arms would come out and the hands would strangle me, so I sat on the stairs. Something old and familiar in me wants to be heard and expressed. Something wants my attention.

Winter 1961

Jack Kennedy was president, but Daddy still wasn't happy and he was yelling at Mommy already and I wasn't even asleep yet. I sat up in bed to see if the closet door was still shut. I left the light on so the monsters would be content to stay in there all night. I could see the yellowish sliver slicing into the room from the corner below the door. The door was shut, and the light was on. I slipped out of bed and stepped into my blue fluffy slippers. Linda always got pink stuff, for girls, and I got the blue stuff. Blouses, sweaters, slippers, bathrobes. That was fine by me. In my blue slippers, I put on my blue robe and stepped off the carpet onto the cold hardwood floor, creeping in the dim nightlight-lit room to the desk. I picked up the desk chair, moved it over to the closet, and propped it against the door under the knob. Safer.

But still, shouting came from the living room. Mommy was crying. I couldn't stand it, and I knew there would be monsters under the bed anyway, so I decided to go sit in the hall and listen. But I didn't understand what they were fighting about and I was afraid to lean against the walls, so I sat in the middle of the second stair and leaned against the top one.

I heard Mommy and I felt sorry for her and I decided to kill Daddy for her, or at least beat him up. I went up the stairs and down the hall to their bedroom and into Daddy's big walk-in closet, where he kept his golf clubs. I pulled one out. Shaking, I steadied the bag. The seven-iron came out in my hands. I walked out of the bedroom and down the hall to the stairs and got about halfway down. I made a pledge in my mind to Mommy: "If he hurts you, I will come in there and kill him, Mommy." I sat there, listening to their fight, until I fell asleep.

When I awoke, it was quiet and cold. I took the golf club with me and crawled back into bed. The house felt like a tunnel. It was quiet the way things are in a movie right after the scary part. I held the seven-iron close, under the blanket. In the morning, I put it back in Daddy's bag and no one was the wiser. I didn't have to kill Daddy that night after all. But was I too cowardly to do it, to save Mommy? I felt like I had let her down. Maybe I should have done something. I wished Linda still slept in this room.

—

Entering a therapeutic conversation is a great relief. I feel supported, as though we have literally put a support under me. It takes a burden off my mind to know that I have a partner working with me. In fact, I feel slightly elated for several weeks afterward. Therapy gives me insights into hidden emotions and how they can trigger panic. I see that I could have used silence like a hideout to avoid dealing with difficult emotions. Grief, certainly, and fear. And maybe some hurt feelings.

Silence is a mysterious but welcoming friend. It took me years of practice to be able to get through the noise to the quiet, but once you get in there and hang out in it, it's possible to relax and get comfortable. As the experience of deep quiet registers in your nervous system, you learn to access states of calm when you need them. I wonder if this is something you could learn as a child, a way of breathing and listening to your own body's inner silence, to calm yourself. Someone would have to teach you. Maybe I will teach my grandchildren, should I ever have any. The thought is heartwarming. My attention follows the breath easily now into silence.

But I've been hiding out in this silence. Its protective blanket is nurturing, but I've been using it to press out other unwanted voices, feelings, and needs. That can't be good. Feelings need a voice. I'd be better off listening to them than waiting for suppressed feelings to take over my throat and vocal cords, sending out distress signals. Have I really suppressed something to the point of fueling panic? If so, I am using a pattern I learned in childhood to make myself—my feelings—disappear. If I've been trying to kill myself off to save Linda, that's a crazy, self-negating plan.

Therapy happens in an atmosphere of trust. You come and talk, and the first thing that happens is that you experience being seen and heard. This lightens your heart, and that invites back into play anything you keep out of awareness. For me, old secrets, buried regrets, and other unfinished business creep back into my awareness. I've created a healing space in my life, and there is a waiting list for my attention. I have to sort things out week by week. I write and write in my journals. I never really reconciled myself with that situation where I . . . I never really closed the chapter on breaking up with . . . And how long have I been afraid to stand up for myself? When did that start?

Things that need to heal come to mind. I make little sketches of all the parts of my psyche that are shifting to healthier, freer states. I draw a timeline of significant life events. I find a storage closet within me with little boxes labeled things like "Difficult Experiences," "Regrets," "Ungrieved Losses," "Things Blamed on Me," "Mistakes I've Made." These need some healing attention.

A lot has happened in the thirty-plus years since I allowed myself the healing atmosphere of therapy. Here I am again, receiving the gift of letting another person listen deeply to me, someone who can help me spot old ideas, wacky thinking, and cognitive distortions. Reframing gives me mind-opening new perspectives on challenges that I successfully met and even conquered. Despite setbacks, I did it all my way. I raised my daughter through college, had a good career in high tech, stayed sober and sane, walked through hard times, and showed up for myself and my family. I've lived my values. My life is one I can be deeply grateful for. Everything is really going so well.

But I also discover that I have some deeply embedded self-negating reaction patterns. My independent, self-defined lifestyle is the living opposite of my mother's, yet, I must admit, I struggle with feelings of victimhood and self-pity. I saw the way my mother was treated and instead I tried to be assertive, but I took on a self-negating base note. I find it difficult to speak for myself. I sometimes feel powerless, somehow a victim of certain situations.

Self-diminishment is opportunistic; it attacks wherever it finds a weakness. Envy of a friend's new car can start a streak of self-doubt or confusion. *Why didn't I save my money for something nice like that?* A coworker's comment could send me into turmoil of embarrassment: "It's cute how you wear that blue eyeliner every day." *Am I doing it wrong? Is it a bad color? What could she possibly have meant?* Perhaps I could avoid shame if I tried harder or disappeared better. Self-negation keeps demanding, all the while eroding your well-being until you feel like you're dragging heavy chains.

I leave JoAnn's office feeling as if we went into the basement, tore all the neatly packaged and labeled boxes off the shelves, and threw everything all over the place.

It feels like everything is all over the place, but I'm really just noticing the habitual reactive patterns in my psyche. The more you bring to awareness, the more you're aware of. Now that I can see these patterns when they arise, what can I do with them? I have two tools: the Confronter and the Witness.

The Confronter is about changing a behavior. I'm willing to challenge the reactive pattern by confronting and changing my behavior. If I find myself, for example, holding down my own voice, I confront that. I find a way to speak at least some part of my voice.

The Witness is about listening and observing the experience of the pattern. The Witness lets the pattern be fully heard the way a parent listens to a hurt child. What does it have to say? What does it feel like when it says it? You get into Witness mode and let yourself be aware of the qualities of the experience. The presence that witnessing brings to your woes helps to melt them.

A friend and I once had a disagreement about the score of the NBA playoff series. I was looking right at the television displaying the score, but my friend insisted on a different score. I actually looked it up in two other places before I had the confidence to assert that the score was, in fact, the set of numbers displayed on the television. Here's the Witness intervention: Witness what's present when the unwillingness to speak up occurs. There's a hesitancy to assert the score—what is that? I am receding, pulling back. I can feel myself retreating, negating my own experience. This is the exact way in which I cut myself off. Observing this, my heart goes out to me. And that is healing, just presence without judgment. That releases old patterns. A few more rounds of presence, and that unwillingness will have a hard time sneaking up on me. The Confronter will just say, "No, here's the real score."

LOVE THE FEAR
Santa Cruz
Winter 2017-2018

When you face any opponent, it's smart to get as real as you can. Your assumptions will be instantly tested. A fantasy that my superior speed will rescue me from a well-timed one-two-three combo might not serve me well. What do I really need to do to protect myself? Probably keep the gloves up and the feet moving—no shame in that. And look again: Where are the real openings in her defense that I can exploit? Does she leave her face open when she jabs? Does she drop her guard when she kicks?

If I enter a fight with fear, that fear clogs my system with cortisol, and that affects my access to energy, clarity, memory, and speed. My mind will be occupied with half-formed fearful thoughts that block access to what I really need. I won't notice when she drops her guard. If I can't channel fear into clean aggression without anger, I'm going to be relating to my fear or my anger energy, instead of to the punches, and that will totally distract me from the fight. I need to get that out of my way so I can focus. It's the same with old patterns. If one rises up—maybe it makes you discouraged, lonely, judgmental, self-critical, ashamed—you want to relate to it effectively so it doesn't crowd your choices.

It's really the same thing with a self-concept. Apparently, being self-aware necessarily includes feeling your "self," and *that* feeling is colored by the self-concept you have stored in your whizzing brain. A self-concept *feels* like a solid, real person, but it's really a bunch of ideas cobbled together, based on very young reactions and strategies. I want my self-concept to be tuned to reality, instead of to unconscious patterns established decades ago. To free it from the grip of old patterns, I've got to refresh any old ideas.

With a renovated self-concept based on fresh data about what's going on, I could have more of me available to respond to what's actually happening. I could be more able to listen to informed urgings rising from the 90 percent. If a right roundhouse gets launched, my front leg will go up for the block *if* I am loose and attentive. If I'm tight and anxious, afraid of the next move, I'll never react with the block on time. That is the fact: When you are out of sync with reality, you suffer.

But we don't know what reality is, and there's the trouble. There are different ways to look at what is real. Are we talking about physical objects, social constructs, economic facts, psychological experiences, or spiritual insights?

We know only the tiniest amount even about physical reality, comprising all those three-dimensional bits floating in space and clicking their way through time. Our body and brain have only the data sent to our nervous system, which are most often just some light waves indicating color, maybe a scent molecule that drafted upstream. Sometimes a sound wave strikes the eardrum or data on temperature or hardness reaches nerves in the skin. A summary of this data reaches the cognitive centers and enters awareness. "Ah, the steaming warm scent of coffee!" This scant evidence is what we've been calling "reality." But that's not a tenth, even a thousandth, of reality. There is so much more going on in a moment.

We are not separate objects moving around in space-time. The outer world is not just the static picture we learned about. A more modern description of ourselves in our physical world is that we are integrated energy quanta interacting incessantly in a collection of flickers that creates and warps space-time while it occurs, as everything interacts with everything else in the quantum equivalent of "six degrees of separation" at every moment. And that's just the physical realm of the body. The mind is far more capricious, energetic, and changing.

Where in all this is what you could call reality? What's a girl supposed to tune her self-concept to?

Here, beating in my own chest, I feel not the joy of my own heart, but fear and distress. I write to my Zen friend. "I went with my older sister to get a bone marrow biopsy. The ledge we are walking is so narrow. I want to be present for her, but I find my mind filled with its own anxieties. I feel useless when all I have is my own baggage."

"Be present for your own fear," he writes back. "Meet that fear with love. When you meet your fear, you are facing a fact: Life is uncontrollable." This is hard to take in. "Take it in. Whatever you can deeply say yes to, you are no longer controlled by. When you feel fear, say yes: 'Yes, I am willing to be afraid.' You'll see that your love is giving you courage to free yourself from your own resistance."

Reality must include all of what's arising, and the reactions, and the awareness that is willing to be afraid. My friend is saying that the reality to be present with, that I can tune to, is whatever is actually arising now, not as a thought but as an experience. Say yes to the present experience. Even if it is unwelcome.

My key to saying yes to whatever is actually present is willingness: willingness to receive what's coming out of the depths, somehow; willingness to listen; willingness to hang out with discomfort and be comfortable with that while the inner 90 percent works things out.

Willingness is risky; it puts your old ideas to the test. It suspends the tight grip you usually have on your safe worldview. You might decide to let go of old stories that could be blocking the flow of more intelligence. If you do get the old unconscious patterns and stories out in the open, you could have access to more knowledge about reality and more insight about how to relate to things.

Willingness is a very powerful tool and ally for this kind of transformation. I first learned about this trick in therapy back in the 1980s. "I can't do it," I'd complain. "My stomach just gets tied up in knots, and I can't think."

"Are you willing to be willing to make the request?" JoAnn would say. We'd go through this same conversation on different topics: asking for a raise, a date, a commitment.

"Yes, I am willing to be willing . . ." I would eventually say every time. I could be absolutely certain I could not take the risk of applying for a new position. I was not even willing to face the possible rejection. But was I willing to be willing? Was I willing to someday be able to face the risk so I could move forward in life? Yes. My attitude would shift just that little bit it needed to shift to alter the trajectory. That would open a pathway beyond my recalcitrant fears. Thus, I slipped past my resistance and headed toward flat-out willingness.

I throw the I Ching. I have found this to be a very helpful little insight gadget. I do this as a way of getting past my thoughts to the wisdom beneath. I do this in the spirit of honoring mystery. I make no claim to understand the history, literature, language, poetry, or mysticism of the I Ching. I merely love Thomas Cleary's reading and use it to illuminate my labyrinthine travels.

I do this in a very simple way: I contemplate a question about which I have some definite intuition. In this case, I have a strong feeling that working at the cognitive level with JoAnn is the right thing to do and is worth my investment of time, money, and attention. But it is a demanding commitment. Is it the right investment for me? I get a feel for both sides of the story—a feel in both my psyche and my body. Then I ask the question "Am I on the right track?"

I take six quarters loosely in my palm. I tune in to the intuitive layer of mind, where I contemplate, "Am I on the right track?" I toss the coins loosely. Then I set them down in a column. I just let my fingers lay the coins out and keep my head out of it.

Heads represents a solid line; tails is a broken. The first three coins are tails, tails, tails. Broken, broken, broken. *Earth.* The next three are heads, heads, tails. Solid, solid, broken. *Wind.* I have thrown Hexagram 46, Rising Up: earth over wind. This reading suggests upward movements guided by great wisdom. It is very developmental, which means there is the potential for great growth. It suggests that the situation is ripe for transformation, but genuine expertise is needed. Hexagram 46 is, I read, a symbol of spiritual maturation into clarity and love, but the seeker should not proceed alone. She should speak to a knowledgeable and trustworthy person. Good heavens— could it be clearer? It's a good time to grow with help from an expert. I feel like a seedling in springtime, comforted with watered compost, stretching in the morning sun.

THRIVING

ONE DAY AT A TIME
Santa Cruz Mountains
Spring 2018

Therapy is a disruptive and enriching process. It's about trying to understand my own experience more deeply and incorporating more of my unconscious life into my awareness and self-concept. I have to disrupt my currently cherished views and attitudes to get new insight.

At the tail end of sixty-six, I am less interested in protecting my viewpoint and more interested in real freedom. I am open to seeing what's really going on under the covers, and because I have a trustworthy therapist I can just get on with the work. In the next six months, we open up and transform the ways I experience shame and the ways I devalue myself. I come to see how I cut my own self off from my own flow of love, creativity, and peace.

In our weekly chats we discover I am often the first one to do things to minimize myself. It turns out, I see with dismay, that in situations when I *feel* unheard or insignificant, I undercut myself before a put-down can actually happen. This puts me in the victim mode. The good news is, since I am doing it, I have the power to change things. Week by week I learn to shift out of victimhood and speak up for myself.

We unearth the internalized misogyny I inherited that has been hiding within me. I see how hard it has been for me to respect women, how I've been socialized to look up to men instead. With surprise I cop to lingering homophobia that still colors my self-concept. I recall that I was the last of all my friends to support gay marriage—it took the support of the straight community for me to finally acknowledge I deserved the full rights of citizenship.

I'm getting in touch with my power to stand up and speak for myself. I'm willing to be responsible and to be happy even if I must confront inner shame and fears. I practice forgiving and embracing myself. I discover I am not an idiot, though I've made a few dismal choices. I am not my mistakes, my shame, my anger, or my humiliations. I begin to feel more real, more whole. I aspire to embrace all of me, all the bright and dark moments. What a relief.

Therapy helps me spot, attend to, and release old ideas. There are old ideas that I am not lovable or that intimacy is always a dangerous risk; that my time and attention are less important than someone else's; that there's something broken about me that I want to hide from others.

As problems often do, these notions weaken as I confront them. Just being aware gives me some space and leverage I can use to move toward freedom.

After a few months of therapy work, I've stopped going to the gym so often. Jill and I are working out for thirty to forty-five minutes at home in the mornings. I do light jogging, weights, and boxing combos. To spar takes more commitment than I currently have. I'm working on my inner body, so the outer body will just have to accept a less demanding regime. I miss the exuberance, but training at the gym used to be a four-hour ordeal, including prep and travel, warm-up and cool-down, class and recovery. Now I have that time for journaling, for walks with Zoey in the woods, cooking, friends, and poetry. I'm reading a couple of books on the structure of poetry and have started writing some of my own.

Today, there is a witness function in my psyche. It has a healthy perspective and does not panic; it has access to my other mental resources, like clear thinking and feelings of well-being. This witness perspective seems to get its self-concept from the qualities reflected in the silence of meditation: peace, strength, and patience. It is getting stronger. My scrunched-up childhood self is invited into my witness self. I am big enough to include everything. I'm a human mystery, a great reservoir, endlessly embracing.

Whatever arises is okay. I can work with it. Everything seems workable. I'm developing the presence of mind to be present for myself as I am. Old patterns need not take over my parasympathetic nervous system. I can witness them and slowly free myself from them. When we find an old idea, I am willing to confront it and let it go. Some are recalcitrant, like tumors, and need repeated applications of willingness and release. I can do that; I will show up for that. We West family girls have mettle.

I am 100 percent ready to thrive. I intend to let that saturate the layers of myself until all of me is in full alignment.

RASPBERRIES AND STRAWBERRIES

Los Angeles
Spring 2018

Linda's body will never be the same, but it is a wonderful, living, breathing, working body that gives us a Linda. Now her work is in the return journey, recollecting and healing.

Weeks turn to months. Linda inches forward, one day at a time. There are obstacles and difficulties, including some backlash from chemo. Her stomach is off. She loses weight. But her bridge game is on, her chess game is on. Her white blood cell count is low, suppressed purposely by medication. They manage GVH pretty aggressively the first year. Her lungs sustained damage from the trial drugs, but that has improved dramatically. So she is weak and often tired, but her spirits are positive and strong.

In February they reduce the immunosuppressants a little and adjust a few other medications. In a few months, her appetite returns and she begins to forget she is recovering. Her energy has been slowly returning. Her overall well-being surges after Day One Hundred. This is a complete success. She gets untethered from City of Hope and put on a fast track for reduced check-ins at Kaiser.

In March, little Alaia comes for a visit. Linda hasn't been allowed to see her since last summer, just before the end of the trial treatment. Lise and Alaia fly down from their home in Seattle; Lise has work to do in the area, so Rick and Linda will babysit. Fortunately, this week is spring break for Santa Monica High School and Uncle Ari is available to help out every day. Linda and Alaia make up stories and paint their nails. Alaia plays hopscotch with Rick—Grandfather Opa—on the tiles in the backyard. They're like little kids together.

Linda has plans to attend a viewing of a ballet and a dinner with friends. She keeps up at the cancer resource center. The white count goes up. The neutrophil count goes up. Her energy and appetite go up. Her hair is about the same length as mine and looks really cute on her.

I dream that I am weaving a space for heartaches to be heard. Leaving room for yellow regrets and red losses, I weave a basket of vines that were fed by streams. I put in bits of shell and green moss, an old, dead stone the color of resentment, and wild purple spring flowers. Gently packing a glass shard, I wrap it in browning elm leaves. Snowballs from Northbrook. Tiny shoes. I add a pale yellow paper funnel of raspberries, ripening in summer, gathered by a little girl.

I text Linda about raspberries.

Rikki: "Didn't Lise tell Alaia that Nana will be able to visit when the raspberries ripen? I read that raspberries in Seattle ripen in July."

Linda: "Yes! I expect to be there baking pies with her in July."

Rikki: "How's it going?"

Linda: "I am starting to do the stuff I love. This weekend we went to a lecture at the Getty. I am going to a book club meeting this week—bringing dinner!—and away with the group for a long weekend in Tahoe at the end of April."

Rikki: "Congratulations! You are ahead of schedule."

Linda: "Yes. Yes, absolutely."

A week later, I text Linda to see if she has gotten results from her latest blood test. She now goes to a local Kaiser once per month. Yet it seems just yesterday we were discouraged by so many trips to City of Hope. Maybe the transplant gods gave her time off for time served, because she spent six months going to City of Hope before she even started the transplant.

She texts me.

Linda: "I got some results yesterday afternoon. My white count is 7.6. Not only is that in the normal range, it's on the high end of the normal range. Neutrophils, too. Things are just awesome.

Rikki: "Why don't you tell me these things? You know I'm on the edge of my seat. Congratulations!"

Linda: "I'm sorry. It's just that I'm starting to think of myself as not sick. Also, I go to the cancer research center for three wonderful workouts: tai chi, Feldenkrais, osteoball. And, wait for it: Alaia is coming again in May! Also, I don't appear to have any GVH and my vision is good. Saturday during the day I am going to the Huntington Gardens to the bonsai exhibit. I have missed the last two years, and I am very glad to be going again. Also, we have had two days of pouring rain. Weather that I love. When did life get so perfect?"

Rikki: "Oh, let me remind you of that research paper saying that the WBC is best indicator of long-term success."

Linda: I did not remember. That is incredibly wonderful. Thank you for telling me. Yes, I believe I will be eating raspberry pies in Seattle this summer.)-: Tears of joy and emotion, not sadness.

Linda sends pictures of Alaia's visit, and Rick begins to develop a cold. A single or double strand of RNA . . .

April 4, 2018: Linda's sixty-ninth birthday. Linda, aka Nana, sends a text to the family.

Linda: "Today is my birthday—and I just want to say a particular thank-you to Rikki. I am very grateful—for everything. Of course, now I also have a birthday on October 24. Rick is going to be very busy with foot rubs from now on."

Lise: "October 24 is the strawberry birthday, as well as your Day Zero."

Rick: "Strawberry?"

Lise: "Nana's strawberry that Alaia brought back to life and then spread to additional pots on Nana's bone marrow birthday. #useallthemagic"

Rikki: "Wait, what? Is there a plant that was potted on October 24, Day Zero, that is now thriving?"

Lise: "Oh, yes."

Linda: "To sum up: in addition to needing a whole new set of stem cells, I required a great deal of sympathetic magic to recover. Lise had to wear the same earrings every day for a year. Alaia had to bring a dead strawberry plant back to life. Lise and Alaia had to transplant the revived strawberry shoots on the exact day."

Rikki: "Now everyone is thriving?"

Lise: "Yes. Even the strawberry plant is thriving. Even my earrings. It's a very good story."

Linda tells the story to the whole listening family in texts:

Once upon a time (in June 2017, while Nana was in the clinical trial), a little girl discovered an abandoned strawberry pot in her backyard. There had once been a strawberry in it, but now it was just a brown stem and a brown leaf sitting on top of the dry dirt.

Do you know what a strawberry pot looks like, Rikki? It's a large urn kind of thing with many cup-like openings along its side, where runners can put forth new plants.

She had just moved into the house. The strawberry was alive when they moved in, but in the weeks that they were there, just as Nana was hearing that her cancer had returned, the strawberry turned brown and, to all appearances, died.

"I'm afraid it's dead," said Mama.

"Yep, looks dead, all right," said Papa.

"We'll put it in the compost," said Nana.

"I think it needs water," said the little girl.

The little girl watered it with her watering can. When they fed the other vegetables, the little girl was sure to water the strawberry, too. But she was very clear that only she and Nana were allowed to water the strawberry.

Since Nana was in Los Angeles, it was up to the little girl.

"Sometimes plants die," said Mama.

"We can get a new plant," said Papa.

"Don't get your hopes up," said Nana.

"I think it needs more water," said the little girl.

She watered and watered. It was a hot, dry summer. And still she watered.

Rikki (interrupting the flow of texts): "Oh dear, you can overwater sometimes. Did it drink the water? Did it have a leaf? Did it turn green?"

Linda: "Lise will have to tell us the rest of the story, because I got a little sick at the end of the trial, and then it was October and time to start the transplant treatments."

Lise: "Alaia watered and watered. A green leaf appeared. No one could believe it. Well, Alaia could. Then there was another. Alaia kept watering. And another. The strawberry grew and grew. It overflowed the pot. Tendrils of strawberry hung to the floor. It grew and grew."

Lise: "So we took a couple of tendrils and tucked them into a little new dirt. Still they grew. They took root. On October 24, we cut the newly established tendrils away from the mother plant and put them in their own pot."

Lise: "They have been quietly hunkering there all winter."

Happy birthdays, Linda!

Rick comes down with a full-blown adenovirus infection.

THE GATHERING
Santa Cruz Mountains
Spring 2018

I am driving around the lot at the Safeway on Forty-First Avenue, looking for a parking space, when I have a satori-like insight. I tend to think *I* shouldn't have to park far away! There's a thought here, in my head, that says *I* always deserve a good spot. Those crummy spots are for other people. Abruptly, I notice I do the same thing in traffic. I think *I* should not have to sit in lines with everyone else, just because I am me. I'm the type of person who uses the HOV lane. I cheat. I make sudden turns down alleys. I shout at my fellows. It's embarrassing, but there it is.

I become distinctly aware of a general urge to escape the common lot. And behind that there is another layer, of self-protective insistence that *I* be special and superior. Privileged. As with most people, part of me wants to find the wisdom, the wealth, or any other way to avoid the ordinary challenges of being human, like loss, grief, and confusion. Like cancer.

But nowadays, instead of pushing everything away like that, I want to let everything be as it is. Instead of trying to escape some parts of life, I'd rather end the struggle. I want to bring presence to whatever is present. That's all.

I intend to welcome all of me: dark and light, soft and hard, weak and strong. It's okay to admit weaknesses, wounds, and failures. It's good to acknowledge feeling afraid, imbalanced, or uncertain, as well as wise, clear, and focused. I welcome what comes from the depths. I am finding a voice for what has been cut off. I embrace and befriend all of me and invite me to come forward and be acknowledged as my Scar Clan, as Clarissa Pinkola Estés likes to call it. The Scar Clan women could be my deep friends if I welcome them and get to know them. These are the parts of me that have been through stuff and know what they're talking about. I don't need to be afraid of them.

I am calling all of us home to a great gathering. I've got kindness. I've got space. I've got patience. And I've got support: daughter, partner, therapist, a good meditation practice, and a great Muay Thai coach. I have room and resources to engage all the different energies that arise. With my magic integrating power, I, Rikki Stormborn, have gathered a wisdom army.

Just saying this, I come to realize, is courageous and possibly revolutionary. You have to figure out how to love yourself while you reveal these protected inner secrets to yourself and accept the reality and consequences. You have to be willing to break out of any self-imposed prison.

This healing process is not something I can control. It takes its own time and finds its own rhythm. JoAnn still catches me in the act of leaving me out. I'll use dismissive language, unconsciously calling my ambitions "silly." I'll downplay an aspiration or hide it from myself, treating it like an old, punctured volleyball, cheap leather worn to the web. I toss out one or two to show their sad state. JoAnn tosses them back: Is this really how you want to treat your dreams?

As I find my voice, I see how I have held it down. I did it to myself. It's a protective device, but it's out of date and off the mark. Some core part of me waited for permission to be. It waited for affirmation that I am valid. It waited for confirmation of my existence. That had to stop. Just by virtue of seeing it, I changed my relationship to it.

Now that I can see the very subtle ways in which I nullify my own power, its influence will diminish. It can no longer totally sneak up on me. It's a matter of my paying attention and listening and welcoming.

After the transplant, I feel in some weird way that my life is not really my own in the same sense it used to be. Rather, it is part of a great arc that is difficult to see—something larger than a life, something that includes multiple lives of people intimately engaged with me. That destiny seems to be moving us all toward encounters with ourselves. From that point of view, I can be patient with myself. My reactive patterns seem like training sessions in how to spot ignorance, or delusion, or a false story. They show me where I have an old pain that needs to be heard, healed, and released.

I've learned what to do with reactive patterns: I meet them with my full kindly attention. Confront, face, listen to, challenge, attend. Whatever it takes to bring the patterns into presence.

Reactive patterns and old ideas fizzle out on their own in the clarity of being clearly seen. You get rid of their burden by being aware of them and by closely, warmly, kindly observing them. You get to be intimate with yourself. It's not that difficult, really; it's actually kind of fun. This is what Mommy would have wanted me to do: confront my demons, claim my space, set my boundaries, own my life energy.

In front of our house runs a sidewalk bordered by night-blooming jasmine on one side and twenty-five rosebushes on the other. At this time of year, especially after our extended spring rain, the buds are fresh and plump at the ends of long, straight stems, bright with pinks and yellows and reds, purple, white, and apricot. The buds whorl their petals out from their vibrant centers. We'll be able to keep fresh flowers in the house for months.

FIRST COLD AND BEST PET
Los Angeles
Spring 2018

Rick gets a persistent upper respiratory infection from the cold that's been coming down on him. About a week later, on April 11, Linda starts coming down with it. It looks like this little strand of supervirus came from the aquarium in Long Beach, where Grandfather "Opa" Rick took Granddaughter Alaia in March. Uncle Ari, who was along for the aquarium trip, is as sick as Opa. So Linda has picked this up from local schoolchildren, a segment of the population best avoided, if possible.

Friday. Linda's immune system is not quite six months old, like a newborn baby's. There are components whose job is to induce the maturation of B cells and T cells. These components take months to mature in a new immune system. Plus, Linda's immune response is still a little suppressed by drugs to prevent GVH. So we can't expect her to mount much of a defense against the virus. She'll just have to weather the storm. It's coming on like a Category 5.

Saturday: I'm hoping she can get through this, plus the PET tomorrow . . . I ask Rick to check with Dr. Farol at their next consultation. Is Linda's system mature enough to produce B cells that can go out and identify this virus? Can they program an immune response and get a load of T cells armed and mobilized? Or is it too soon for that?

Sunday: Fever glanced toward 101 last night but goes back to 99 by the morning. She gets the PET and puts it behind her. But by midday the temp rises again above the critical level and stays there for a while, so they go into urgent care. After they consult Linda's various physicians, they decide to keep her for observation. By the evening, she doesn't have a high temperature anymore, but the slightly raised temperature is persistent and they have to be very cautious about the possibility of a bacterial infection of the blood. It will take two days to get the culture results, so they keep her hospitalized.

This is the normal way to get through colds and infections in these early months after a bone marrow transplant. It is how they manage Linda as an outpatient. They treat opportunistic infections with antibiotics and don't rely on her immune response yet. "It's another bump on the road, but we're going to ride it out," says Rick. He has remained remarkably cool throughout this. He's gotten used to extreme measures in the past couple of years, but things should slow down now as Linda continues to heal.

Monday: Linda remains in the hospital for observation and prophylactic treatment with antibiotics. She's in a pretty low-risk state as long as she has this medical support. They miss their consultation with Dr. Farol, so we don't know the outcome of the PET yet. I consider the fact that I haven't had any road rage for months.

Tuesday: I wonder if Linda is intimate with death now, the fear of it, the threat of it, the respite from it. Her temperature remains slightly elevated, but tests come back negative for bacterial infection. She has a viral pneumonia, not a big problem. She doesn't feel too much worse than a very bad cold makes you feel. They expect to send her home tomorrow. Does intimacy with death change how you relate to the living moments you still have?

Wednesday: Linda is released in the morning and spends the afternoon in her backyard. Indomitable! The Category 5 has passed through without leaving any long-term damage. After restoration of services and general cleanup, she'll be back on track.

A week later, April 23, Linda and Rick meet with Dr. Farol to review the PET. Results: no activity. This means there is no active cancer in Linda's body. The tumor is dead, the marrow is clean, the new lymph and blood products are made from new cancer-free and cancer-eating genetics. Tomorrow is April 24, exactly six months since the transplant.

Our work here is done.

Here's my checklist, April 24, six months exactly:

- Viable donor!

- Perfect match!

- Get into trial to stay alive until transplant!

- Complete trial!

- Get transplant!

- Transplant takes over 93 percent, but we get to 99 percent!

- No graft versus host (GVH) disease!

- Heal completely—even get through a category 5 head cold and viral pneumonia!

- Kill tumors—clean PET; no cancer present!

Outside my den window, drops of rain have coalesced into clumps that are freezing into tiny balls on the way down. Clackety-clack-clack, they strike the eaves as little ice pellets. My daughter telephones, and I start talking about plans for her commitment ceremony—aka wedding—next September. I am deep into possible catering options when she tells me she's called to ask for help editing a paper. She is in the last two weeks of several years of graduate work to prepare her for practice as a marriage and family counselor. She is practicing already at the clinic at the school. Music still weaves throughout her life; her fiancé is a talented musician pursuing his doctorate in ethnomusicology. She used to sing with the Threshold Choir, an a cappella group for patients in hospice, and currently sings with an Eastern European folk group. I let her know I can look at the paper this afternoon.

Jill is away on a late-season ski trip, it is storming outside, Zoey is asleep under my desk, and I have the afternoon free. Linda texts me that she is going to Seattle to visit her daughter, son-in-law, and granddaughter in early June, a few weeks before the raspberries ripen, but it's been a warm season in Seattle, so perhaps they will be early, like Linda.

Like the seeker at the beginning of this story, I don't know where the pilgrimage is going or where it ends. If I have become intimate with anything, it is myself. I am feeling myself to be connected to a deep well, carried by invisible life streams that protect me, and nourished by rootlines that link me to other lives. I feel the upwelling of myself as voice and energy and happiness. May we all feel the joy of our own hearts beating in our own chests.

EPILOGUE

At one year post-transplant, Linda's marrow shows 100 percent successful acceptance of the grafted stem cells. All her blood products are generated from the new genetics.

At one and half years post-transplant, the doctors announce that Linda is cured. The new immune system has destroyed any lingering cancer cells. She no longer has lymphoma. Her healthy immune system effectively protects her from opportunistic invasion.

ACKNOWLEDGMENTS

I offer heartfelt gratitude to my dear early readers, whose encouragement meant so much, and special thanks to Jill, Jake, and JoAnn. You made all the difference.

ABOUT THE AUTHOR

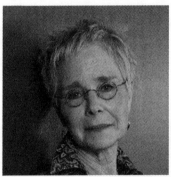

© Reenie Raschke

Rikki West is a birdwatcher, book lover, and student of meditation who started training in Muay Thai at age sixty-two. She took her bachelor's in genetics at the University of California at Berkeley and her master's in integrative humanities at San Francisco State University. Her greatest passion is ideas, and her greatest thrill is understanding a new subject, perspective, or person. Thai kickboxing, journaling, and meditation support her aspiration to awaken as much as possible before her lights go out. Now retired from a thirty-five-year high-tech management career, she is the mother of Lauren Magnolia and godmother of Morgan Lisa and lives in Santa Fe, New Mexico, with her spouse, Jill.

Check out her website at www.rikkiwest.com

SELECTED TITLES FROM SHE WRITES PRESS

She Writes Press is an independent publishing company founded to serve women writers everywhere. Visit us at www.shewritespress.com.

Edna's Gift: How My Broken Sister Taught Me to Be Whole by Susan Rudnick $16.95, 978-1-63152-515-5

When they were young, Susan and Edna, children of Holocaust refugee parents, were inseparable. But as they grew up and Edna's physical and mental challenges altered the ways she could develop, a gulf formed between them. Here, Rudnick shares how her maddening—yet endearing—sister became her greatest life teacher.

Rethinking Possible: A Memoir of Resilience by Rebecca Faye Smith Galli $16.95, 978-1-63152-220-8

After her brother's devastatingly young death tears her world apart, Becky Galli embarks upon a quest to recreate the sense of family she's lost—and learns about healing and the transformational power of love over loss along the way.

A Different Kind of Same: A Memoir by Kelley Clink $16.95, 978-1-63152-999-3

Several years before Kelley Clink's brother hanged himself, she attempted suicide by overdose. In the aftermath of his death, she traces the evolution of both their illnesses, and wonders: If he couldn't make it, what hope is there for her?

Change Maker: How My Brother's Death Woke Up My Life by Rebecca Austill-Clausen $16.95, 978-1-63152-130-0

Rebecca Austill-Clausen was workaholic businesswoman with no prior psychic experience when she discovered that she could talk with her dead brother, not to mention multiple other spirits—and a whole new world opened up to her.

Don't Leave Yet: How My Mother's Alzheimer's Opened My Heart by Constance Hanstedt $16.95, 978-1-63152-952-8

The chronicle of Hanstedt's journey toward independence, self-assurance, and connectedness as she cares for her mother, who is rapidly losing her own identity to the early stage of Alzheimer's.